The Detox Diet

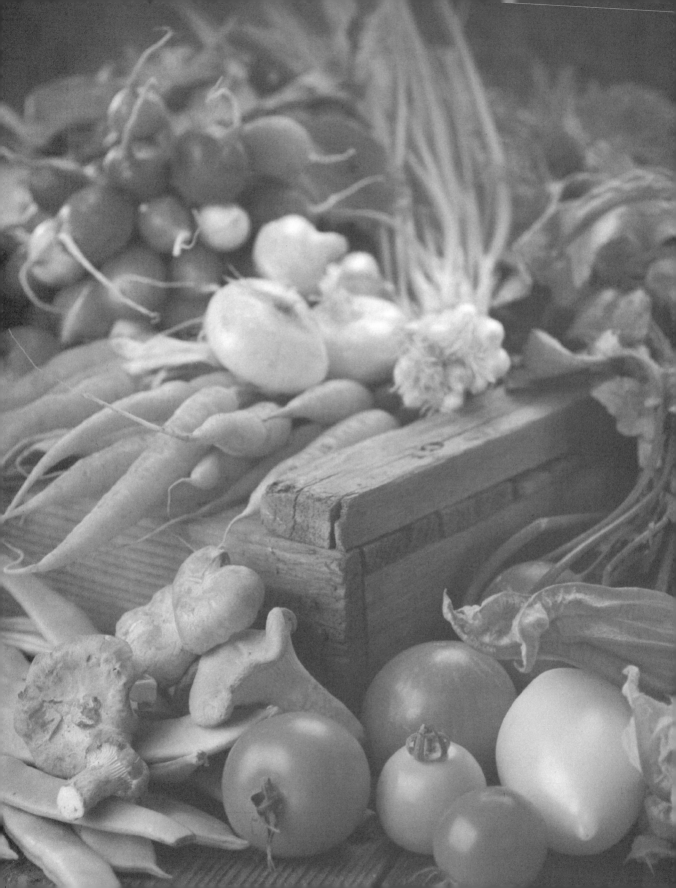

The
Detox Diet 3rd Edition

The Definitive Guide for Lifelong Vitality with Recipes, Menus, and Detox Plans

ELSON M. HAAS, MD, The Detox Doc®
with Daniella Chace, MSN

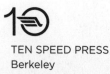

TEN SPEED PRESS
Berkeley

The information contained in this book is based on the experience and research of the author. It is not intended as a substitute for consulting with your physician or other health-care provider. Any attempt to diagnose and treat an illness should be done under the direction of a health-care professional. The publisher and author are not responsible for any adverse effects or consequences resulting from the use of any of the suggestions, preparations, or procedures discussed in this book.

Published in the United States by Ten Speed Press, an imprint of the
Crown Publishing Group, a division of Random House, Inc., New York.
www.crownpublishing.com
www.tenspeed.com

Previous editions of this work were published in the United States as *The Detox Diet* and *The New Detox Diet* by Celestial Arts, Berkeley, in 1997 and 2004.

Ten Speed Press and the Ten Speed Press colophon are registered trademarks of Random House, Inc.

Library of Congress Cataloging-in-Publication Data
Haas, Elson M., 1947–
    The detox diet : the definitive guide for lifelong vitality with recipes, menus, and detox plans / Elson M. Haas, Daniella Chace.—3rd ed.
        p. cm.
    Summary: "Guides readers through the detoxification process and follow-up cleansing programs for those struggling with addictions to sugar, caffeine, nicotine, and alcohol"—Provided by publisher.
    Rev. ed. of: New detox diet / by Elson M. Haas, with Daniella Chace. 2004. 2nd ed.
    Includes bibliographical references and index.
    ISBN 978-1-60774-325-5 (pbk.)
1. Nutrition. 2. Detoxification (Health) I. Chace, Daniella. II. Haas, Elson M., 1947–
New detox diet. III. Title.
    RA784.H32 2012
    613.2—dc23

                        2012000938

ISBN 978-1-60774-325-5
eISBN 978-1-60774-326-2

Printed in the United States of America

Cover design by Toni Tajima
Interior design by Katy Brown

Third Edition

10 9 8 7 6 5 4 3 2

Dedicated to you and your healthy habits,
which will lead to great lifelong health.
Enjoy more from less.

"You've been provided with a perfect body to house your soul for a few brief moments in eternity. So, regardless of its size, shape, color, or any imagined infirmities, you can honor the temple that houses you by eating healthfully, exercising, listening to your body's needs, and treating it with dignity and love."

—DR. WAYNE DYER

"I will feed and nourish you, if you just love me."

—MOTHER EARTH

Contents

Acknowledgments

Dr. Elson Haas wishes to acknowledge:

First, I wish to thank **my readers** for supporting *The Detox Diet* (1996) and *The New Detox Diet* (2004), for being aware of the importance of detoxification, and for spreading the word about this needed healing therapy.

Thank you **Bethany Argisle** for your continued contribution to my writing career and for keeping your awareness on the pulse of the earth. And thank you for your writing touch, personal stories, and many ideas for this book.

A very special thank you to **Daniella Chace** for your spark, motivation, and support for this new edition, and for your writing contributions, recipes, and smooth communications. You are a great and knowledgeable nutritionist.

Thank you **Dr. Sondra Barrett** for your invaluable research and critical thought on all the revised text, especially on the statistics and costs associated with substance abuse.

Thank you also **Ten Speed Press**, **Crown Publishing**, and **Random House** for your support of the Third Edition—especially **Veronica Randall**, for your expert guidance and editing, and **Toni Tajima** and **Katy Brown**, for your cover and book design, and **Sara Golski**, for taking over and completing this new edition.

Thanks also to **Drs. Franz Morrell** and **Alexander Wood** for the nutritional concepts that helped formulate my original Detox Diet.

Daniella Chace wishes to acknowledge:

Dr. Elson Haas—thank you for being a great inspirational teacher, with a forward vision in helping our teens and youth prevent disease through detoxification and good health practices.

A heartfelt thank-you to our editor, **Veronica Randall**—your awareness and intuition as to what is relevant to our readers today has been invaluable in our revisions, as has your ongoing encouragement to share our personal experiences.

I'm grateful also to **Sara Golski** for your exceptional editing skills and attention to detail.

Thank you to my health-conscious mother, **Linda Landkammer**, for your wisdom and loving support.

A special thank-you to **Matias Booth** for your recipe testing and research.

Ten Speed Press, **Crown Publishing**, and **Random House**, thank you for supporting the revised edition of this book as a solid source of detoxification information for more than a decade.

Thank you **Richard Calcagno** for introducing me to Dr. Haas all those years ago.

Preface

From Dr. Elson Haas

When I did my first fast using the Master Cleanser in 1976, I never thought cleansing and detoxification would become so important in my life and career. Well, today it makes perfect sense given our exposure to toxic chemicals and pollutants in our air, water, and food. Nowadays, the topic of detoxification is even more relevant, and detoxing programs have become increasingly popular among people young and old.

Although there are many detox books in the marketplace, I believe the one you have in your hands is the most basic, sensible, and easy to follow. Its practical guidelines have been an empowering tool in my medical practice for the past thirty years, with literally thousands of patients experiencing positive and measurable benefits.

Originally published in 1996, *The Detox Diet* has been used by many other physicians and natural-health practitioners. In fact, I connected with nutritionist and author Daniella Chace because she was using my book with her individual clients

and detox groups and realizing consistently excellent results. I believed the addition of her experiences and expertise could improve the book, and I invited her to contribute to the 2004 edition. We are again working together with our newly updated and expanded 2012 edition, in which we are very excited to include a chapter dedicated to teenagers—a new group to inform and inspire toward healthier living.

The detoxification process is an individual path, followed moment by moment, season to season. You may find it helpful and motivating to keep a journal of your experiences during this process. Take the time to reflect not only on the physical changes you experience but also on the psychological and emotional changes that occur on your path toward lifelong vitality.

So, give it a try! You have nothing to lose—except unhealthy habits and excess weight! Let *The Detox Diet* be an important next step toward being your own best doctor.

From Daniella Chace

When *The Detox Diet* was first published in 1996, it was a small book with big ideas in an era when the medical and naturopathic worlds were still divided. Finally, here was a book written by a medical doctor that addressed the underlying causes of disease, that wasn't focused on treating symptoms with medications or invasive procedures, and that was passionate about the value of nutrition. *The Detox Diet* was a seminal book that brought sound information and clear guidance to an audience who was ready to embrace both. Today, countless clinics and health spas provide detox workshops, juicing books have became popular, and neighborhood natural food stores have grown into mainstream supermarket giants.

In my own practice in Sun Valley, Idaho, more and more clients became interested in detoxing, until, eventually, it seemed everyone in our little mountain town showed up at my door for a three-week cleanse sooner or later—and many of them brought *The Detox Diet* with them! And supplementing Dr. Haas's program with my own recipes, menu plans, and nutritional supplement recommendations became routine.

As I became increasingly focused on toxicology and detoxification, contact with Dr. Haas seemed inevitable, and to my delight, one of my class participants, Richard Calcagno, was also a patient of Dr. Haas. He suggested a merging of our materials would make an even more comprehensive book for those who couldn't attend a workshop. I called Dr. Haas—and *The New Detox Diet* was born.

We believe *The Detox Diet, Third Edition*, is the most comprehensive detox guide to date. It includes the most current research, many new recipes, a new chapter for teens, and much more.

We hope you enjoy the detox experience, and we are honored to be your guides in this valuable process.

Elson Haas, MD, The Detox Doc®
and Daniella Chace, MSN
January, 2012
pmcmarin.com
haashealthonline.com
daniellachace.com

Part One
RENEWAL

So many problems in our society come from excessive use of food, chemicals, and drugs. Abuses and addictions touch almost every person's life. I realize these habits are as much a part of our social and cultural upbringing as they are our responses to dealing with the stresses of family, school, work, our local environment, and society at large. Food choices are especially a challenge for so many overweight and obese people, an expanding and significant issue for many of us across all age groups, from young to old. Truly, finding the right, supportive, and balanced diet is a dilemma for most everyone.

I don't want you to feel bad or weak or self-conscious if any of these potentially destructive habits applies to you. I know the struggle between light and dark, between picking up that bag of cookies or chips, that cup of coffee or glass of wine or pack of cigarettes—and the desire to stop. I also know it is an incredible challenge to change anything, particularly to stop any addiction we have relied upon for many years. For most of us, our habits serve us well until they don't, and most of them undermine our health in a variety of ways.

I have seen consistently that clearing our substance habits can be done with greater attentiveness to our actions, with a gathering of our willpower, and with the support of our family and friends. I have also seen that it is very difficult to change our habits if we are not also willing to deal openly with emotions and other adversaries that may block healing.

I do want to inspire and motivate you to change. **The first principle and action for improving your health is to eliminate destructive habits.** Even if you cannot believe that you can do without your substances completely, at least consider an abuse break and observe the change. Try a day or a week without caffeine, alcohol, or sugar, replacing them with a new habit of drinking water, walking, or swimming. See how you feel. Remember, breathe deeply.

All addictions are ultimately self-destructive (some may hurt others as well, such as alcohol and smoking). When you change that dynamic to self-care—through your internal healing process as well as by following the lifestyle and nutritional guidelines I describe in this book—you will begin to better serve your body and move your life toward its higher potential. As you develop more nurturing and supportive habits—eating good food, exercising regularly, learning to cope with stress, and developing motivating attitudes—I know you will experience greater vitality, more positive relationships, and overall improved health.

Good luck on your journey.

CHAPTER ONE

Why Detox?

DETOX: HOAX OR HEALING?

I have used the process of detoxification and the information in this book for more than thirty-five years for my personal well-being as well as for many thousands of patients, with even more people benefiting from the process since the publication of the first edition of this book. Of course, there are many other practitioners who guide and observe people through similar processes of elimination diets, detoxification programs, and juice cleansing and have thousands of positive anecdotes. We still do not have much research that backs up what we see. It is challenging to first study the multidimensional programs people typically employ and then compare them with placebos or different diets. This research gold standard (double-blind, placebo-controlled study) is much easier when evaluating one substance, like a new medicine.

Really, we are talking here about a complete lifestyle shift, as with diet, exercise activities, and attitudes. Thus, to skeptics, it's all a bunch of talk. "Prove to me that it works," states a scientific researcher. I say, "Let me put you on a program and we'll see how you feel and look. And we can study your blood chemistry, such as your cholesterol level (especially when it's high), or monitor your blood pressure. Many aspects of your health will get better, with many side benefits." I know when people make lifestyle and habit changes they often have improved health results.

Still, it's difficult to study whole programs for improved health. Here, experience and anecdote might be a better gold standard.

THE DETOX CONTROVERSY

The broad topic of detoxification diets is filled with controversy, the main arguments against them being that there's no scientific proof detox diets work, and that they are not needed at all because the liver and kidney do a fine job clearing the body of its toxins. In addition, the opponents of detoxification claim these diets cannot be maintained for long periods of time without doing major harm, that they are a scam to sell useless products and procedures. For doctors who have been trained to treat disease, the whole approach to the nutritional management of disease—actually the prevention or reversal of disease—is a hard pill to swallow because it suggests that conventional Western medical training is both deficient and incomplete. This is why I veered into natural medicine after my own medical training—because I felt my education to date had taught me almost nothing about health and what was needed to keep the body fit. (I feel this is also a deficiency in public school education. Yet, that has been changing over the past decades.)

The concepts and practices of detoxification are an integral part of natural medicine. Detoxification is done by every cell in the body, and almost every organ system helps in the body's waste removal. The human body continually detoxifies itself, yet when it is stressed or overloaded, the body may not be able to keep up and then may create a symptom or other form of "communication" about the imbalance.

In these cases, the body tries to rebalance itself by flooding the connective tissues with acids, which eventually can cause more inflammation and aging. This is one of the basic ways we stress our bodies. The discussion of acid-alkaline diets and body states is an essential understanding for overall health and I believe will be the medical understanding in the future when it comes to viewing health and disease.

Detoxification is a process, not really a diet. To me, the truth about helping our bodies detoxify is that it allows us to learn about our individual bodies, incorporate a process to simplify our intake for a short period of time, and then develop a healthier lifestyle understanding. When we eliminate certain foods and substances, we have the opportunity to see, experience, and learn how our bodies respond. This is invaluable in the process of healing, and individualizes it. Thus, your own personal experience proves or disproves the process to you, and maybe to your doctor if the doctor believes every patient's medical treatment is ultimately an experiment or experience. To me, this is the right way to practice medicine, through direct experience and observation with an eye on safety first, as in "First, do not harm," a key Hippocratic principle of the oath taken by medical doctors. I believe that detox programs, when done appropriately for the right people, may prevent chronic illnesses, reduce existing problems, and improve health and vitality.

Medical research is costly and, unless you are testing a patented product, there is no money for the proofs the opponents and skeptics ask for. To me, the proofs are in how people feel and look after they have completed a round of cleansing/detoxification and have changed their habits. These programs also commonly help people increase their awareness of foods and substances that don't support their health. Finally, when someone is attempting to eliminate addictive substances like tobacco or alcohol, having a diet plan to support the process is useful and necessary.

Thus, think of detoxification as something you can do to help yourself feel better and learn what works for you in terms of your individual eating and intake program. Can you handle coffee, sugar, or alcohol, or does even a little bit throw you off or reduce your vitality? When you consume these substances every day, you may not be able to sort that out. That's why I encourage you to take breaks—a week to a month—to eliminate what you take for granted and do every day, see whether you feel better after a few days, and then incorporate them again (one at a time) to experience how you really feel.

WHAT IS TOXICITY AND DETOXIFICATION?

Toxicity is a great concern in our modern world for literally everyone. No one can avoid environmental exposure. Threatening our health are powerful chemicals, air and water pollution, electromagnetic waves, noise pollution, radiation, and nuclear waste. We ingest new chemicals, use more drugs, eat more sugary and refined foods, and abuse ourselves daily with stimulants and sedatives. Cancer and cardiovascular disease are on the rise; arthritis, allergies, obesity, and skin problems are also rapidly increasing; and a wide range of symptoms such as headaches, fatigue, pains, coughs, gastrointestinal problems, immune weaknesses, sexually transmitted diseases (STDs), and psychological distress like depression are being seen by physicians in record numbers. Although a connection between increased toxicity and increases in diseases is obvious, it is important to understand how toxins occur so we can avoid or eliminate them from our lives.

Toxicity primarily comes from two basic areas—external and internal. We can acquire toxins from our environment by breathing them, ingesting them, or being in physical contact with them. Most drugs, food additives, and allergens can create toxic elements (from reactions and by-products) in the body. In fact, any substance can become toxic when used in excess.

Internally, the body produces toxins through normal everyday functions. Biochemical and cellular activities generate substances that need to be eliminated. These unstable molecules, called free radicals, are biochemical toxins and are considered a common factor in chronic disease. When these biochemical toxins are not counteracted or eliminated, they can irritate or inflame the cells and tissues, blocking normal functions on all levels of the body. Microbes such as intestinal bacteria, foreign bacteria, yeasts, and parasites can produce metabolic waste products that we must handle. Even our thoughts, emotions, and stress (including stress caused by the daily news) can increase biochemical toxicity. The proper elimination of these toxins is essential. **Clearly, the healthy human body can handle certain levels of toxins; the concern is with excess intake, excess production of toxins, or a reduction in the elimination processes.**

A toxin is basically any substance that creates irritating and/or harmful effects in the body, undermining our health and stressing our biochemical or organ functions. Chemicals and metals (lead and mercury) can interfere with the many sensitive enzymes that catalyze most cell functions and affect overall cell and body health. Toxin irritation may also result from the side effects of pharmaceutical drugs or from unusual physiological patterns. The irritating chemicals, or free radicals, from the use of both prescribed and recreational drugs can also cause tissue degeneration. Negative "ethers," psychic or spiritual influences, and the stress from bad relationships, negative thought patterns, and emotions can also have toxic effects on our body.

Even if we are living in a basically healthy way, toxicity still can occur when we ingest more than we can utilize and eliminate or breathe polluted air.

Homeostasis refers to balanced bodily functions. This balance is disturbed when we feed ourselves more than we need or when we abuse specific substances. Toxicity may depend on the dosage, frequency, or potency of the toxin. A toxin may produce an immediate or rapid onset of symptoms, as many pesticides and some drugs do, or it may have long-term effects, as when asbestos exposure leads to lung cancer.

When our body is working well, with good immune and eliminative functions, it can handle everyday exposure to toxins. However, when we are stressed or not sleeping well, we may not be able to handle even our normal amount of toxins. This could also be a cyclical function, like so many body functions; sometimes our bodies are strong detoxifiers and other times they are weaker.

BEFORE YOU BEGIN

As a physician, I am fascinated by the complexity, subtlety, and diversity of individual health habits—specifically, the combinations of various substances we imbibe and ingest. The spectrum of these substances includes the components of our diet (foods, drinks, chemicals), supplements (nutrients, herbs, and homeopathic remedies), drugs (prescription, over-the-counter, and recreational), and pollutants (herbicides, pesticides, hydrocarbons, and petrochemicals). These all are part of our possible choices and have effects on our life and health, both present and future.

Some questions we might ask ourselves:

- How do we develop our preferences?

- When do our preferences become needs?

- Why do our needs become addictions?

- Why do some of us become addicted while others of us can stop on our own? Is it inherent or learned?

Personality, upbringing, and environment influence our personal choice of substances. In exploring these concerns about abuse and the way it affects our health, I have developed a specific orientation and program for initial healing and detoxification. This process has evolved over my nearly forty years as a naturally based, general health practitioner.

My overall understanding of symptoms and disease integrates both Western linear thinking and naturopathic approaches to health and illness. Problems with the body and mind often arise from either **deficiency** (when we are not acquiring sufficient nutrients to meet our bodily needs) and/or **congestion/toxicity** (when our intake is excessive or we ingest something that is particularly irritating). Congestion can arise from both reduced elimination function and an overconsumption of food or substances such as caffeine, alcohol, nicotine, refined sugar, and chemicals from medications to home cleaners to freeway fumes. It's clear that noises and smells affect us as well and those of us

who are more sensitive to these issues can find ways to protect ourselves from these exposures.

People who are deficient in nutrients may experience problems such as fatigue, coldness, hair loss, or dry skin. They need to be nourished with wholesome foods (and supportive relationships) that aid healing. However, **congestive problems are more common in Western, industrialized countries.** Many of our acute and chronic diseases result from clogged tissues, suffocated cells, and subsequent loss of vital energy. Frequent colds and flus, cancer, cardiovascular diseases, arthritis, and allergies are all consequences of congestive and inflammatory (often tied together) disorders and, eventually, too many antibiotics, other medicines, and surgeries that result from these problems. These medical problems may be prevented or treated through a process of cleansing, fasting, and detoxification. These approaches represent different degrees of an overall process that reduces toxin intake and enhances toxin elimination, making way for health and healing to occur.

All of the programs contained in this book combine aspects of these fasting and detoxification/cleansing processes. Herein, there are specific programs for dealing with **Sugar, Nicotine, Alcohol, Caffeine, and Chemicals (recreational drugs and prescription medications)—what I call SNACCs.** In each program, I discuss the physiological actions and reactions involved, the hazards

HEALTH REVIEW: DO I NEED TO DETOX?

Rate your potential for toxicity (with the following topics, activities, and medical symptoms) OR rate the prevalence of your habits and medical symptoms to help determine whether detoxification will be of benefit to you now.

PERSONAL HEALTH REVIEW

Score each answer on a scale from 0 to 3. The key is:

- 0 = I **avoid** a substance or food, or I **never** experience a symptom or condition.
- 1 = I **occasionally** use a food/substance, or I **occasionally** experience a symptom/problem (< 3 x week).
- 2 = I **frequently** use a food/substance, or I **frequently** experience a symptom/problem (> 3 x week).
- 3 = I use a food or substance on a **daily** basis, or I experience a symptom or problem **daily**.

The higher your score, the more likely you will benefit from the Detox Diet and detoxification.

SNACCs: Score (0 to 3)
____ SUGAR
____ NICOTINE
____ ALCOHOL
____ CAFFEINE
____ CHEMICALS
____ Prescription medications
____ Over-the-counter medications
____ Recreational drugs
____ Artificial sweeteners

____ **TOTAL SNACC SCORE**

Foods:
____ Dairy products
____ Wheat and bread products
____ Fish
____ Beef
____ Smoked or organ meats
____ Nonorganic food
____ Soda
____ Restaurant dining

____ **TOTAL FOODS SCORE**

Medical Symptoms:

___ Headaches
___ Allergies
___ Sinus congestion
___ Cough or mucus
___ Skin rashes
___ Acne outbreaks
___ Painful periods (dysmenorrhea)
___ Back pain
___ Joint pain
___ Tendonitis or fasciitis
___ Other pain
___ High blood pressure
___ High cholesterol
___ Digestive upset
___ Constipation
___ Irritable bowel syndrome
___ Bad breath
___ Fatigue
___ Insomnia
___ Anxiety
___ Depression
___ Diabetes, adult

___ **TOTAL MEDICAL SYMPTOMS SCORE**

Other Factors:

___ Computer use
___ Cell phone use
___ Television
___ TV news
___ Driving or commuting in a car
___ Stressful relationships
___ Perfume or cologne
___ Chemical deodorants
___ Chemical cleaners at home
___ Chemical exposure at work
___ Dental amalgams

___ **TOTAL OTHER FACTORS SCORE**

TOTALS FOR EACH:
___ SNACCs
___ FOODS
___ OTHER FACTORS
___ MEDICAL SYMPTOMS
___ **TOTAL (all categories)**

UNDERSTANDING YOUR SCORE

60+	Detox NOW!
45 to 60	Clearly benefit from detox
30 to 45	Consider some detox
< 30	Great going!

and ill effects of the substance, and the methods for handling and clearing these adverse habits.

The beginning of the process for healing our abuses requires motivation from within to change unwanted habits. This often requires us to address the underlying emotions that may perpetuate the problem. A good counselor or therapist or a compassionate positive friend can be helpful to support this healing process; and remember, for real healing, it takes what it takes for the worthwhile experience of truly getting better. Overall, we must create a workable plan and gather our willpower to begin. The Detox Diet and other purifying programs discussed throughout this book alkalize the body, help us feel better quickly, and lessen feelings of withdrawal. Drinking good water, getting vigorous exercise, and taking specific nutritional and herbal supplements also support the detoxification process.

A few simple tenets of natural medical practice may help clarify for you this book's approach:

1. The primary cause of disease is the accumulation of unnecessary wastes that are not properly eliminated, resulting in poison retention, cellular dysfunction, and subsequent health problems.

2. Your body is designed to support optimal function. Listen to its signals.

3. Given the proper environment, your body has the power (and likelihood) to heal itself and return to its normal healthy state.

Patients and physicians do best when oriented to live and practice with a commonsense approach that first looks at lifestyle as a place to promote rejuvenation, then to natural therapies, and finally to pharmaceutical drugs and surgery, which are appropriate when a situation is acute or severe or if natural therapies are not working. Lifestyle factors include diet, exercise, good sleep, stress management, and attitudes.

Motivation is helpful for our behaviors and outcomes. Are we motivated from a crisis or do we seek a better, healthier future?

Natural therapies include nutritional supplements, herbs, homeopathic remedies, and hands-on healing such as massage, osteopathy, and chiropractic care. Nutritional awareness and practice aid you in both preventing disease and recovering health.

Put simply, **the key to maintaining metabolic balance is to maximize nutrition and both minimize and eliminate toxins.**

The goal is to place your health and that of your family back into your own hands. In fact, so much of your health is up to you. Take the initiative to do what you can to be vital and healthy. It is really worth it!

CHAPTER TWO

General Detoxification and Cleansing

THE PURPOSE OF THIS CHAPTER is to understand the importance of detoxification; discuss ways to support the elimination of excessive toxins, mucus, congestion, and disease; and prevent the buildup of further toxicity. The cleansing process encourages our immune system, liver, and blood to handle the elimination of toxins and abnormal cells generated by the body. This may even help reduce our risk of cancer, which I believe regular, healthy detoxification does.

Our body handles toxins by neutralizing, transforming, or eliminating them. For example, many of the antioxidant nutrients, such as vitamins C and E, beta-carotene, zinc, and selenium may neutralize free-radical molecules. The liver helps transform many toxic substances into harmless agents the blood carries away to the kidneys; the liver also sends wastes through the bile into the intestines, where they are eliminated. We also

---

OUR GENERAL DETOXIFICATION SYSTEMS

Gastrointestinal—liver, gallbladder, colon, and the whole GI tract
Urinary—kidneys, bladder, and urethra
Respiratory—lungs, bronchial tubes, throat, sinuses, and nose
Lymphatic—lymph channels and lymph nodes
Skin and dermal—sweat and sebaceous glands and tears

---

clear toxins by sweating, either from exercise or from heat; our sinuses expel excess mucus when congested; and our skin releases toxins daily, which can also cause reactions we may experience as skin rashes.

Mental detoxification is also important. Cleansing our minds of negative thought patterns is essential to health, and physical detoxification can aid this process. Emotionally, a physical detoxification helps us uncover and express hidden frustrations, anger, resentments, and fear, and replace them with forgiveness, love, joy, and hope. Many people experience new clarity of purpose in life during cleansing processes. A light detoxification over a couple of days can help us feel better; a longer process and deeper commitment to eliminating certain abusive habits and eating a better diet can help us change our whole life. Detoxification is part of a transformational medicine that instills change at many levels. Change and personal evolution are keys to healing.

An important topic to consider in *The Detox Diet* is electromagnetic toxicity, which has become so commonplace in these modern times with our daily exposure to computers, cell phones, and televisions, plus radiation exposure from airplane travel and medical testing. In some ways, this persistent electrical interaction with our bodies may alter our sensitive cellular, biochemical, immune, and neurological systems. Our bodies are electric (electromagnetic), and clearly our cells and nerves function and communicate electrically. It

Excess Detox?

I want to express some concerns about overelimination or overdetoxification, which I occasionally see. Some people go to extremes with fasting, laxatives, enemas, colonics, diuretics, and even exercise and begin to lose essential nutrients. This can cause protein or vitamin and mineral deficiencies. So, although congestion from overintake and underelimination is a more common problem in this culture, excessive detoxification can be a concern as well.

makes sense that our bodies pick up and can be altered by this interaction. Thus, in addressing toxicity and detoxification, we should be aware of these electromagnetic issues as well.

Many people have addictive behaviors when it comes to their relatives and loved ones, and these are difficult to identify without taking a break and stepping outside the day-to-day interactivity. With the process of detoxification through the use of detox diets, there are often increased insights into personal feelings and attitudes toward others and our work as well. As we will mention later, our relationships can go through some detoxification and changes when we follow a detox program.

WHO SHOULD DETOXIFY?

Almost everyone needs to detoxify and rest the body from time to time. Some of us need to cleanse more frequently or work more continually to rebalance the body. Cleansing or detoxification is but one part of the trilogy of nutritional action (the others being building or toning muscle, and balancing or maintaining the body). A regular, balanced diet devoid of excess necessitates less intensive detoxification. Our bodies have a daily elimination cycle, mostly carried out at night and in the early morning up until breakfast. When we eat a congesting diet higher in fats, meats, dairy products, refined foods, and chemicals, detoxification becomes more important, particularly to those who eat excessively and to those who overeat at night.

Our individual lifestyles provide clues for deciding how and when to detoxify. If we have any symptoms or diseases of toxicity and congestion, we will likely benefit more from detoxification practices. It is like a vacation for the body and especially for the digestive tract.

Common toxicity symptoms include headaches, fatigue, congestion, backaches, aching or swollen joints, digestive problems, allergy symptoms, and sensitivity to environmental agents such as chemicals, perfumes, and synthetics. Dietary changes or avoidance of the symptom-causing agents is usually beneficial. However, it is important to differentiate between allergic and toxicity symptoms in order to determine the appropriate medical care. This Detox Diet program, as well as fasting and juice cleansing, can all be genuinely

---

SIGNS AND SYMPTOMS OF TOXICITY

Headaches	Immune weakness*	Depression*
Joint pains	Environmental	Sexual dysfunction*
Coughing	sensitivity/allergy	Fatigue*
Wheezing	Sinus congestion	Skin rashes*
Sore throat	Fever	Hives
Tight or stiff neck	Runny nose	Nausea
Angina pectoris	Nervousness	Indigestion
High blood fats	Sleepiness*	Anorexia*
Backaches	Insomnia*	Bad breath
Itchy nose	Dizziness*	Constipation
Frequent colds*	Mood changes*	Menstrual pain
Irritated eyes	Anxiety	

*These symptoms could also result from deficiency.

helpful in reducing allergy symptoms; however, allergies present a dynamic subtly different from that of toxicity. The key is to figure out and avoid the allergens from our environment and from our foods. The detoxification programs in this book will help us avoid almost all of the typical allergens we get from our foods and habits.

Detoxification and cleansing can contribute to the healing of many acute and chronic illnesses that result from short- or long-term congestive patterns. Detoxification and cleansing also benefit people with addictions to numerous substances. However, because withdrawal symptoms can commonly occur with the detoxification of many drugs, I recommend conscious, informed management of the detoxification process.

Detoxification is also an important component in treating obesity. Many of the toxins we ingest or make are stored in the fatty tissues; hence, obesity is almost always associated with toxicity. When we lose weight, we reduce our body fat and thereby our toxic load. However, during weight loss we also release more toxins and need to protect ourselves from nutrient depletion with extra supplementation, including drinking more water and taking

---

PROBLEMS RELATED TO CONGESTION / STAGNATION / TOXICITY

Abscesses	Gout	Prostate disease
Acne	Obesity	Menstrual problems
Boils	Infections from:	Vaginitis
Eczema	Bacteria	Varicose veins
Allergies	Virus	Diabetes
Arthritis	Fungus	Peptic ulcers
Asthma	Parasites	Gastritis
Constipation	Worms	Pancreatitis
Colitis	Uterine fibroid tumors	Mental illness
Hemorrhoids	Cancer	Multiple sclerosis
Diverticulitis	Cataracts	Alzheimer's disease
Cirrhosis	Colds	Senility
Hepatitis	Bronchitis	Parkinson's disease
Fibrocystic breast	Pneumonia	Drug addiction
disease	Sinusitis	Tension headaches
Atherosclerosis	Emphysema	Migraine headaches
Heart disease	Kidney stones	Gallstones
Hypertension	Kidney disease	Sexual dysfunction
Thrombophlebitis	Stroke	

additional antioxidants to balance these toxins. Exercise will also promote the loss of excess pounds and help further detoxification.

Of course, not all of these problems are related solely to toxicity, nor will they be completely cured by detoxification. Still, many conditions are created by nutritional abuses and can be alleviated by eliminating the related toxins and following a detoxification program.

WHAT IS DETOXIFICATION?

Detoxification is the process of either clearing toxins from the body or neutralizing or transforming them, which can also help clear excess acidity, mucus, and congestion. Fats (especially oxidized fats and cholesterol), free radicals, and other irritating molecules act as toxins on an internal level. All of this can increase body inflammation, which is the basis for so many chronic diseases. Functionally, poor digestion, colon sluggishness and dysfunction, reduced liver function, and poor elimination through the kidneys, respiratory tract, and skin all increase toxicity.

Detoxification involves dietary and lifestyle changes that reduce the intake of toxins while improving elimination. The avoidance of chemicals from food or other sources, including refined flour and sugar products (so plentiful everywhere), caffeine, alcohol, tobacco, and drugs, helps minimize the toxin load. Drinking extra water (purified) and increasing fiber by

including more fruits and vegetables in the diet are also essential steps.

A more rigorous detox diet is one made up exclusively of fresh fruits, fresh vegetables (either raw or cooked), and whole grains (both cooked and sprouted), plus some raw seeds or sprouted seeds or legumes eaten fresh in salads. No breads or baked goods, animal foods, dairy products, alcohol, caffeine, or nuts are used. This diet keeps fiber and water intake up and hence, helps colon detoxification. Most people can handle this quite easily and make the shift from their regular diet with only a few days of transition. Others prefer a brown rice fast (a more macrobiotic approach) for a week or two, eating three to four bowls of rice daily along with liquids such as green or herbal teas. Vegetable and miso soups can also be consumed.

An even deeper level of detoxification involves a diet consisting solely of fruits and vegetables—all cleansing foods. The green vegetables, especially the chlorophyllic and high-nutrient leafy greens, support purification of the body and gastrointestinal tract. Fresh juices can also be consumed.

A raw foods diet is fulfilling for many people, yielding high energy and quality nutrition. It utilizes sprouted greens from seeds and grains such as wheat, buckwheat, sunflower, alfalfa, and clover; sprouted beans such as mung or garbanzo; soaked or sprouted raw nuts; and fresh fruits and vegetables. Cooked food is not allowed with this diet, as eating foods raw

CASE STUDY: CAROLYN, AGE 52, MARRIED, MOTHER, BUSINESSWOMAN

I have been fighting the weight loss game for forty years, always with conventional and not so conventional diets, from Weight Watchers to pills to fad diets, and always with the same results. I would lose twenty pounds and gain back forty. By the time the year 2000 came along I was weighing in at 265 pounds, and for my height of 5' 7" that was a lot. I decided to go with my husband to the Preventive Medical Center of Marin, where Dr. Haas was conducting a group on something called "The Purification Process." What have I got to lose? (Ha!) At the first meeting, we discussed the different levels of changing my habits and getting the results all overweight or unhealthy people seek—long-term weight loss and feeling and being healthier. Our group was embarking on Dr. Haas's Three-Week Autumn Detox. I first cleaned up my sugar and caffeine habits, the basis of the Detox Diet. Then, I followed the recommendations I found in Dr. Haas's *The False Fat Diet* (Ballantine Books, 2000) on reactive foods, like cow's milk and wheat products. We would even include fasting, the more extreme part of the process, and since I had done that many years before, I thought, why not? This whole process worked for me and I started to lose (let go of) weight and the feeling of heaviness. I also felt lighter and more alive. The first couple of days of the fasting part were hard, but I stuck with the Master Cleanser (page 53), and all the water, oh, the water.

For the first time I learned what detoxifying really meant. I got off my usual three to four soft drinks a day habit along with all the junk food I had been consuming for years. You could say I was a "junk-food junkie." I continued the fast for nine days, and I really could not believe how good I was feeling. The aches and pains I usually had

in my legs at bedtime were gone, I was thinking more clearly, and, most important, I was losing weight. For years I had been taking medication for hypertension, which I assumed I would be on for life. However, that life was changing. With Dr. Haas's guidance and support, I began to decrease my dosage and eventually went off my meds as my blood pressure kept staying low. It's now several years later, and I have not needed to take any medicine since shortly after starting the detox program.

After the fasting, I went on the False Fat elimination program and stayed off the sugar, wheat, dairy, and junk foods. I followed the Detox Diet as well, and to this day, I make this my lifestyle.

From this new way of eating (and I still enjoy my foods, maybe even more because I know I am really nourishing myself), it has been about two years and I have lost a total of ninety pounds. I exercise five days a week, which is something I had not done for more than twenty-five years. I have never felt better, and my skin has improved tremendously. I have a retail jewelry business, and my longtime customers come in and ask me, "Where is the lady who used to work here?" They clearly don't recognize me, or the new me, and that makes me feel great.

I continue to this day to stay free of the sensitive seven foods (wheat, cow's milk, soy, sugar, corn, eggs, and peanuts) and detox two to three times a year. And I have the tools to rebalance myself just in case I do mess up or go off my diet for a day or two. Then I take a few days to get back into my program and feel better again almost immediately. I am completely off any medications and take only supplements. And most important, I continue to love living life.

CASE STUDY: CINDY, AGE 44, NURSE

I have a condition called paroxysmal atrial tachy-cardia (PAT), which is when my heart suddenly beats very fast, about two hundred beats per minute. My cardiologist recommended a proce-dure called a cardiac ablation where they locate the irritable heart cells and destroy them with electrical impulses. It is an invasive surgery and very expensive. I was very scared.

I started to investigate all my options. I was motivated to change my diet and my lifestyle. I knew the gradual weight gain of fifty pounds over five years was not helping my heart, so I tried many diets. I have been a nurse for more than twenty-five years and felt empowered to make better choices, so I stopped all caffeine, got my cholesterol down to 185 from 210, and did lots of stress management like yoga, energy work, and chanting. I felt better, but the arrhythmia continued.

I tried so many diets. I was drinking fresh-squeezed carrot juice every day. I was unable to get the weight off. I started to blame myself. I felt like such a failure. I knew something was missing. That's when I met Dr. Elson Haas.

At our first appointment, I told him about my heart and my weight. He said very boldly, "From everything you've told me, I think you have a can-dida (yeast) problem." I replied, "No, I don't think so. I work full time and am not a chronic fatigue–type person." He asked, "Do you have bloating after your meals?" I said, "Yes." He said, "If we can clear you of the candida, your heart may work better by lowering the yeast toxins in the blood. Let's have you send off blood and stool tests."

Three weeks later I was stunned to learn I had 4+ *Candida albicans* (that's maximum) growing in my intestines, and elevated antibodies in my blood suggesting immune reactivity. He told me

to read chapters one, two, and three in his very straightforward book, *The Detox Diet*. He gave me a list of supplements to start on and a sheet on how to do the anti-candida diet. He had explained how all my good intentions of drinking carrot juice were just like feeding sugar to the yeast. I was encouraged because now we had found a pos-sible culprit. I now knew where to put my energy. Yet still, I didn't know what results to expect.

Within two weeks of following Dr. Haas's rec-ommendations I had lost ten pounds, and I felt great. By ten months I lost a total of forty-eight pounds. Now my heart is regular and strong. My emotional health is so much better. I met the man of my life and at age forty-five I got married for the first time. My PMS is so much less severe, and we are enjoying trying to get pregnant.

I am grateful to Dr. Haas for his precise diag-nosis. His wisdom and ability to integrate new ideas into his medical practice truly makes him a pioneer in the health-care field. He found the one piece of the puzzle no one else cared to find. Instead of blaming myself, I was able to clear the yeast from my body, and this made a huge dif-ference. Plus, I made very positive changes in my diet, and this has provided other benefits in terms of better energy, stable moods, and quality sleep. The lifestyle changes took some getting used to, but the hard work paid off.

Today I am able to tolerate foods I used to be sensitive to, within moderation. And when I do feel bloated or gain weight I go right back on my program and feel better.

maintains the highest concentrations of vitamins, minerals, phytonutrients (plant-based special nutrients and many acting as antioxidants), and important enzymes—especially when we chew our food well. Many people feel this is their best diet, and I think it can be supportive over quite some time if it is properly balanced.

Detoxifying and healing diets are also available, specifically for problems such as yeast overgrowth or food allergies. In chapter 7, we include an anti-yeast diet and an anti-allergy (hypoallergenic) diet. They involve aspects of detoxification and rebalance.

The liquid cleanses or fasts move beyond the alkaline detoxification and fruit-and-vegetable diets. Juices, vegetable broths, and teas can be used to purify our bodies during fasting. Miso soup, made from a paste of fermented soybean, also provides many nutrients and supports

colon function by aiding the intestinal bacteria. Spirulina (an algae powder) or other blue-green freshwater algaes like chlorella can also be helpful to fasters who experience fatigue by providing amino acids for protein building (add to juices for best flavor) as well as B vitamins and minerals.

Water fasting is more intense than fasting with juices and often results in more sickness and less energy. Paavo Airola, one of the country's pioneers of fasting in America, states in *How to Get Well*: "Systematic undereating and periodic fasting are the two most important health and longevity factors." Consuming fresh, diluted juices from various fruits and vegetables can be a safe and helpful approach for many conditions. Furthermore, specific juice regimens may be used beneficially by people for whom water fasts are contraindicated. Juices help eliminate wastes and dead cells while building new tissue with

---

LEVELS OF DIETARY DETOXIFICATION

- Basic diet
- Reduce toxins daily: ingest fewer congesting foods and more nourishing ones (see chart on pages 20–21); for example, decrease drugs, sugar, fried foods, meats, and dairy. Eat more fresh fruits and vegetables. Takes one to seven days.
- Fruits, vegetables, whole grains, seeds, and legumes
- Raw foods
- Fruits and vegetables
- Fruit and vegetable juices
- Specific juice diets, Master Cleanser, apple, carrot, and greens, and so on (see chapter 4)
- Water

the easily accessible nutrients. See more in chapter 4.

The key to proper treatment is to individualize your program. Take into consideration your general health, physiological balance, energy level, and current lifestyle to set up the right program for you. If you are unsure, start with the basic diet and gradually intensify toward juice fasting and see how you feel. Take a couple of days for each step, and, if you feel fine, move to the next level as described in the box on page 18.

Detoxification therapy—particularly fasting—is the oldest known medical treatment on Earth and a completely natural process. Of the thousands of people we have worked with who have used cleansing programs, the majority of them have experienced very positive results. We believe this detoxification process to be a practical and effective health-care therapy in the twenty-first century and an important first step toward healing our planet.

RANGES OF DETOXIFICATION

Moving to a less congesting diet, as shown in the chart on pages 20–21, will also induce and support healing.

The effects of dietary detoxification vary. Even mild changes from our current eating plan will produce some responses, while more dramatic dietary shifts can produce a profound cleansing. Shifting from the most congesting foods to the least— eating more fruits, vegetables, grains, nuts, and legumes and less baked goods, sweets, refined foods, fried foods, and fatty foods— will help most of us detoxify somewhat and bring us into better balance overall.

Maintaining the same diet but adding certain supplements such as fiber, vitamin C, other antioxidants, chlorophyll, and glutathione (mainly as amino acid L-cysteine) can also support detoxification. Herbs such as garlic, red clover, echinacea, and cayenne may also stimulate detoxification, as can saunas, sweats, and niacin therapy (see chapter 6 for more discussion of supplements for detoxification).

Simply increasing liquid intake and decreasing fats and refined flour and sugar products will improve elimination and lessen toxin buildup. Increased consumption of filtered water, herb teas, fruits, and vegetables while reducing fats (especially fried foods, red meat, and milk products) will also help detoxification. A vegetarian diet may also be a healthful step for those with some congestive problems. Meats and animal products like eggs and milk products, breads, and baked goods (especially refined sugar and flour) increase body acidity and lead to more mucus production as the body attempts to balance its chemistry. The more alkaline vegetarian foods enhance cleansing. The right balance of acid and alkaline foods for each of us is, of course, an important key.

ACID-ALKALINE BALANCE—A KEY TO HEALTH AND LONGEVITY

The concepts of congestion/toxicity and deficiency/depletion relate to the duality of balance that also includes the acid-alkaline poles. The general ideas about illness and health expressed in this book relate to the relative states of acidity, and the congestion, irritation, and inflammation that come from this overly acidic imbalance. The acidity in the body tissues arises from the over intake of too many acid-causing foods (see the chart below). This acidity causes the breakdown and degeneration of tissues over time. The Detox Diet of steamed vegetables and fresh fruits, water, and alkaline drinks helps better balance the body and decrease these acid wastes. The body then lowers its inflammatory and pain states and begins to feel better, more flexible, and more youthful.

The acid-alkaline balance is crucial to what scientists call the *biological terrain* of the body, or the state of the body's tissues and functions. I believe it is this terrain that affects whether or not we are healthy and can fend off most diseases. Parasitic, fungal, and other infections are secondary to imbalances of the terrain; diet, stress levels, and other aspects of lifestyle can profoundly influence the terrain. Because animal products, refined foods, nuts, and seeds are more acidic in their chemical makeup, they create acid residues when metabolized in the body. They contain higher amounts of the minerals phosphorus, sulfur, chlorine, and iodine, while the more alkaline-generating foods typically contain higher levels of calcium, magnesium, potassium, and sodium. These include most high-water-content fruits

---

DETOXIFICATION RANGE

Most Congesting ←

many drugs	fats	sweets
allergenic foods	fried foods	milk
organ meats	wheat, baked goods, refined flour	eggs
hydrogenated fats	red meats	pasta
		fish/poultry

More Potentially Toxic ←
More Acidic* (generally)

* The above chart is not exactly acid-alkaline, but suggests a general tendency for the foods and substances on the left to be more acidic, and toward the right, more alkaline.

and vegetables, as well as some grains and almonds.

Over time, the consumption of an animal product–based diet creates an acidic state of the tissues, with chronic toxicity shown through congestion, irritation, inflammation, and degeneration. The results of this process are the many painful and terminal diseases people experience as they age. That's why body and dietary alkalinization and detoxification are so vitally important to long-term health.

Over the years I have had patients follow their overall pH levels—assessing their blood, urine, and/or saliva, and then monitoring any changes, especially in urine and saliva—to chart their course of healing. There is clearly a strong correlation between body fluid pH and the level of health or disease of the individual. If our tissues accumulate more acid, the kidneys

attempt to release acid and withhold bicarbonate, which makes the blood more alkaline.

Acid states appear in people with acute and chronic inflammatory and pain syndromes, congestive disorders that include recurrent infections and allergies, and the degenerative diseases such as cancer, cardiovascular problems, and diabetes. Once these chronic degenerative diseases have set in, they are more difficult to treat or correct. When I have been able to assess and rebalance an individual's biochemistry, I have seen the lessening of symptoms, the halt of disease progression, and even the reversal of some conditions—and I have experienced this with thousands of patients.

The specific Detox Diet, originally referred to by me as the Alkaline Detoxification Diet, is a smooth and long-range transitional healing program for many

			Least Congesting
nuts	rice	roots	fruit
seeds	millet	squash	greens
beans	buckwheat		herbs
oats	potatoes		water
			More Detoxifying More Alkaline*

people and problems. It is the great biochemical balancer for the person consuming the typical Western diet, a diet I have worked diligently to change both personally and professionally. Educating my patients about this healing Detox Diet is an important priority in my practice.

WHEN IS THE BEST TIME TO DETOXIFY?

Whenever we feel congested, our first step is to follow detoxification procedures fine-tuned to our specific needs. When I start to feel congested from too much food, people, or activities, I will feel better if I can exercise, sauna or steam, drink loads of fluids, eat lightly, take vitamins C and A, and get a good night's sleep. If you feel like your colon requires further cleansing, take stimulating, laxative-type herbs.

Our bodies have natural cleansing cycles when they want a lighter diet, more liquids, and greater elimination than intake. This occurs daily (usually from the night until midmorning, about an hour after we wake) and it may occur for longer periods weekly and more commonly for a few days a month. Women, in particular, are aware of this natural cleansing time with their menstrual cycle. In fact, many women feel better both premenstrually and during their periods if they follow a simple cleansing program of more juices, greens, lighter foods, and herbs during or around their menses.

CASE STUDY: TOBIN, AGE 30, CAMERAMAN

Tobin lives in Sun Valley, Idaho, and came to one of Daniella's Spring Detox classes in hopes of regaining energy and vitality. He came away with some unexpected results.

He cleaned the toxins from his home and eliminated chemicals and toxic foods from his diet. Tobin explained, "I was surprised to find that as my body became cleaner, my mind became clear, and I no longer tolerated emotional frustrations. I felt like I had to rid myself of 'toxic emotions.'" He went to the extent of facing up to his boss and expressing some long-repressed feelings.

Tobin also felt the cleansing work he did and the fast acted as a catalyst that helped him clarify his relationship with food. "I was eating when I wasn't even hungry. I saw this clearly. I had been feeding my inner child junk food as a treat, and now I see that emotional process going on and I can intervene. I did intervene."

Annual seasonal changes can be stressful for some people—at these times, it's a good idea to reduce external demands as much as possible, lower consumption in general, and pay attention to how our inner world mirrors the outer world. When winter turns to spring and when summer turns to autumn are ideal times for yearly detoxification. I suggest at least a one- to two-week program at these times. In spring, we may eat more citrus fruits, fresh greens, juices, or the Master Cleanser (page 53); while in autumn we may dine on harvest fruits, such as apples or grapes, and seasonal vegetables. An abundance of fresh fruits and vegetables are appropriate for summer; and whole grains, legumes, vegetables, and warming soups best simplify our diet in winter.

The sample yearly detox program provided on pages 24–25 is designed for a basically healthy person who eats well. It is not appropriate for people with heart problems, extreme fatigue, underweight conditions, or poor circulation (those who experience coldness). More complete, in-depth fasting programs may release even greater amounts of toxins (see chapter 4). Releasing too much toxicity can make sick people sicker; if this happens, increase fluids and eat normally again until you feel better. People with cancer need to be very careful about how they detoxify, and often they need regular, quality nourishment.

Note: Fasting should be done only under the care of an experienced physician (usually one who is naturopathically trained, which could include MDs, DOs, NDs, DCs, and more). All people should avoid fasting just prior to surgery and then wait four to six weeks before beginning a fast or any strenuous detoxifying. Pregnant or lactating women should avoid detoxification, though they can usually handle mild programs that basically eliminate unhealthy substances while they eat healthy foods; any consideration of detoxifying during pregnancy should be reviewed with the guidance of a qualified practitioner. Also, people can detoxify by improving their food quality with nourishing fresh foods while avoiding junk and high-calorie, low-nutrient choices as well as by trying an elimination diet (such as avoiding wheat and dairy or soy and sugar) to see how they feel and then re-challenge themselves with each food to see whether it causes any problems.

WHERE CAN WE DETOXIFY?

Many people may think that they need to go away on retreat to do any detox or diet changes. Yet these changes don't usually stick when they return home. I believe (and see from my regular detox groups) that doing detox programs at home and living our normal lives allows us to make changes which we can carry forward in the weeks and months following the program

During basic, simple detoxification programs, most of us can maintain our normal daily routine. In fact, energy, performance, and health often improve. For some, the detox process may produce headaches, fatigue, irritability, mucus congestion, or aches and pains for the first few days. Any of the symptoms of toxicity may appear; however, usually they don't. Symptoms that have been experienced previously may recur transiently during detoxification; sometimes it is hard to know whether or not to treat them. Because my approach to medicine is to allow the body to heal itself, I support the natural healing process

SAMPLE YEAR-LONG DETOX PROGRAM

Note: Whether you choose the seasonal or mid-season detox, when buying your fruits and vegetables, look for organic, seasonal, and fresh whenever possible.

SPRING

For 7 to 21 days between March 10 and April 15 (or later in the cold or northern climates) use one or more of the following plans:

- Master Cleanser (page 53).

- Fruits, vegetables, and leafy greens, including blue-green algaes (spirulina, chlorella, blue-green algae).

- Juices of fruits, vegetables, and greens.

- Herbs with any of the above.

- Elimination and food testing can also be done at this time.

The plans can be alternated or can include a 3- to 5-day supervised water fast. Remember to take time for the transition back to the regular diet (about half as long as the fast itself), which hopefully will have changed for the better. (See recipes in chapter 5 and in part 3.)

MID-SPRING

Take a 3-day cleanse around mid-May as a reminder of or return to healthy habits and as an enhancer of food awareness.

SUMMER

Try 7 days of fruits and vegetables and/or fresh juices to usher in the warm weather sometime between June 10 and July 4.

LATE SUMMER

Take a 3-day cleanse of fruit and vegetable juices around mid- to late August.

AUTUMN

Take a 7- to 10-day cleanse between September 11 and October 5, such as:

- Grape fast—whole and juiced—all fresh and preferably organic.

- Apple and lemon juice together, diluted.

- Fresh fruits and vegetables, raw and cooked.

- Fruit and vegetable juices—fruit in the morning, vegetables in the afternoon.

- Juices plus algae such as spirulina, or other green chlorophyll powders.

- Whole grains, cooked squashes, and other vegetables (for a lighter detox).

- Mixture of the above plans, with garlic as a prime detoxifier.

- Basic low-toxicity or elimination diet, with additional herbal program. This could be 2 or 3 weeks avoiding sugar, caffeine, alcohol, wheat and dairy products, as one example.

- Colon detox with fiber (psyllium, pectin, and so forth) along with enemas or colonics.

- Prepare and plan a new autumn diet, enhancing positive dietary habits.

MID-AUTUMN

Take a 3-day cleanse with juices or in-season produce in late October to early November to keep us healthy during the holiday season.

WINTER

A lighter diet, eaten for 7 to 14 days, in preparation for the holidays (or as a detox from them) can be done between December 10 and January 5:

- Avoid toxins and treats; eat a very basic wholesome diet.

- Brown rice, cooked vegetables, miso broth, and seaweed for 7 to 10 days; ginger and cayenne pepper can be used in soups.

- Saunas or steams and massage—you deserve it!

- Hang on until spring!

whenever possible unless the person is very uncomfortable or the practitioner or patient is very concerned.

It is wise to begin new programs, diets, or lifestyle changes with a few days at home. In time, experience will show what works best. Most of us can maintain a regular work schedule during a cleanse or detox program (and we may even be more productive). However, it might be easier to begin a program on a Friday, as the first few days are usually the hardest. Some of us may be more sensitive during cleansing to the stress of our work environment or to chemical exposures. Also, coworkers or family members may provide temptations or challenge our decisions. Having supportive guides or co-cleansers can be a great comfort and source of positive reinforcement when our inner resolve begins to fade. At the end of the first or second day, usually around dinnertime, symptoms like headache and fatigue may begin to appear, and it is good to be able to rest and spend time in familiar, undemanding surroundings. By the third day, we usually feel pretty stable and ready for work.

Still, many people like to start new programs on a Monday, knowing they will do fine, using willpower and positive visualization to see themselves through. People often feel better than ever and are able to accomplish tasks and meet challenges more easily than usual. In fact, experienced fasters may utilize juice cleansing

during busy work periods to improve their productivity; I know this has worked for me. Preparing and planning, clearing doubts and fears, and keeping a daily journal are all useful during this vital process and are crucial to any successful undertaking.

REASONS FOR CLEANSING

Prevent disease
Reduce symptoms
Treat disease
Cleanse body
Rest organs
Purify
Rejuvenate
Lose weight
Clear up skin conditions
Slow aging
Improve flexibility
Improve fertility
Enhance the senses
To be more:
  Creative
  Motivated
  Productive
  Relaxed
  Energetic
  Conscious
  Inwardly attuned
  Spiritual
  Environmentally attuned
  Relationship focused

WHY DETOXIFY?

We detoxify/cleanse for health, vitality, and rejuvenation—to clear symptoms, treat disease, and prevent future problems. A cleansing program is an ideal way to help us reevaluate our lives, make changes, or clear abuses and addictions. Withdrawal happens fairly rapidly, and as cravings are reduced we can begin a new life without the addictive habits or drugs.

We cleanse because it makes us feel more vital, creative, and open to emotional and spiritual energies. Many people detox/cleanse (or, more commonly, fast on water or juices) for spiritual renewal and to feel more alive, awake, and aware. Jesus Christ, Paramahansa Yogananda, Mahatma Gandhi, Dr. Martin Luther King Jr., and many other spiritual and religious teachers have advocated fasting for spiritual and physical health. Some celebrities, such as Willie Nelson and Beyonce Knowles, have talked about their juice-fasting practices.

Detoxification can be helpful for weight loss, although this is not its primary purpose. Cleansing is more important as an overall lifestyle and dietary transition. However, just the simplification of our diet will have some detoxifying effects in our body. Anyone eating 4,000 calories daily of fatty, sweet foods in a poorly balanced diet who begins to eat 2,000 to 2,500 calories daily of more wholesome foods will definitely experience detoxification, weight loss, and improved health simultaneously.

We also cleanse/detoxify to rest or heal our overloaded digestive organs and allow them to catch up on past work and become functionally current. At the same time, we are inspired to cleanse our external life: cleaning out rooms, sorting through the piles on our desks, clarifying our personal priorities, or revitalizing our wardrobes. Most often our energy is increased and becomes steadier as we detox, motivating us to change both internally and externally.

FOOD CHEMICAL EXPOSURE

In Daniella's clinical experience, she has found her clients' symptoms are often associated with toxic exposure. Many people come to her office in search of nutrients to relieve symptoms such as headaches, joint pain, nervous disorders, infertility, and skin conditions. Yet, what she finds is that they primarily need to eliminate rather than add. Toxic food chemicals are often the culprits. Once they eliminate or reduce exposure to chemicals, including hormones, food colorings, preservatives, sulfites, pesticides, and herbicides (with organic foods), they experience a marked reduction in symptoms while regaining their health and vitality.

Although we are exposed daily to chemicals through our water, air, cleaning products, and personal care products, our greatest risk of chemical exposure is through our foods. This is also the area over which we have the most control. If you suspect food chemical reactions are a problem for you, try to avoid them by reading labels and buying organic produce, meats, packaged products, and dairy. Also, when eating in restaurants ask them for more organic foods. If we all begin asking and demanding chemical-free foods and products, we will continue to support the growing and necessary organic industry.

HYGIENE AWARENESS

Proper hygiene inside and outside our bodies and personal environments is one of the four laws of good health, along with eating an alkaline-based diet of wholesome foods, exercising daily, and having proper rest, relaxation, and recreation. Although I believe germs have a harder time causing problems in a healthy body, they do cause certain kinds of problems from mild colds and flu to life-threatening infections. Therefore, do what you can to protect yourself and do not share your germs too freely with others.

HEALTHY HYGIENE HINTS

1. **Wash your hands** several times daily—especially after eliminating, before handling food, after handling animals, when you are sick with an upper respiratory problem (coughing, sneezing, or runny nose), or when you are in close physical contact with others. Also, clean up after a public encounter, such as handshaking, door-opening, or using public phones.

2. **Bathe or shower** at least once daily, more if you are sweaty or dirty, in a clean tub or shower; also, use environmentally friendly hygiene products and cleansers.

3. **Exercise and sweat** regularly to help cleanse your skin and body, and move the lymphatic fluids.

4. **Keep your nails clean** and cut, and clear out dirt and germs that may get under them with hydrogen peroxide or a nailbrush.

5. **Do not put used utensils or your hands into group food.**

6. **Blow your nose** and rinse out your nose and sinuses when you are congested.

7. **Follow safe-sex guidelines,** especially with a new partner.

8. Make sure your diet and activity level facilitate at least one or two **good bowel movements** a day and clean yourself properly afterward.

9. **Keep your kitchen and refrigerator clean;** wash counters and cutting boards regularly. Don't let germs breed in your trash bins—wash them regularly as well.

10. **Minimize your use of and exposure to chemicals** at home and in the workplace. Don't replace germs and dirt with chemicals.

CHAPTER THREE

Gastrointestinal Health: The Guts of Detox

GASTROINTESTINAL FUNCTION AND ECOLOGY (the microbial makeup) are at the core of human health. In other words, our overall health and well-being are influenced by how well we are able to digest and absorb our food, and by the levels of good and potentially harmful bacteria that live in our bowels. The intestinal functions also influence the body's toxin load and in a sense begin the process of detoxification. Cleansing and healing the gastrointestinal (GI) tract (especially the colon) provide a base for effective detoxification, primarily in how well and regularly we eliminate.

The liver has many functions as part of the GI tract, including digestion, metabolism, and detoxification. The liver needs our support with healthy living. Not stressing the liver and giving it some rest helps with both the detoxification processes and the organ's metabolic work.

The statement "We are what we eat and assimilate, and not what we eliminate," is really saying healthy GI tract function is vital to the process of nourishing our bodies and controlling toxicity through elimination, a process that only ends in the colon, yet is done in every cell as well. Furthermore, we must regularly cleanse the intestinal system to effectively detoxify the body. Specific therapies are discussed throughout this book; in this chapter, there is a basic discussion of the GI tract process and its contribution to overall health—a relationship often overlooked in Western medicine.

In this model (which I call Functional Integrated Medicine), the function, ecology, and permeability of the GI tract are crucial to our health. *Dysbiosis* is the term used to describe an imbalance of GI function, specifically related to incomplete food digestion and assimilation, and especially, its microbial populations. Functional Integrated Medicine works with the theory that imbalance in a body system precedes abnormal function; abnormal function precedes symptoms; and symptoms, left unchecked, can precede pathology. This is why the GI tract is assessed for dysbiosis, and particularly for an imbalance in the gut bacteria, as well as overgrowth of yeasts and parasites.

Therefore, to prevent pathology, normal functioning must be restored. This is particularly true of the GI tract, yet is also related to the health of every cell. When this concept of prevention is incorporated into mainstream medicine, we will keep people (and they will keep themselves) healthier longer and prevent disease by evaluating and maintaining proper internal function and environment. Fortunately, this shift in lifestyle approach is gaining momentum around the country.

The digestive process begins in the mouth and continues with the esophagus and stomach, and the small intestine (duodenum, jejunum, and ileum) and large intestine (colon). Proper GI tract function starts with adequate chewing, which is essential for good nutrition and health. Other digestive organs include the salivary glands, pancreas, gallbladder, GI mucous glands, and liver. Salivary enzymes in the mouth begin digestion and the process is continued by hydrochloric acid in the stomach, plus the many pancreatic enzymes that are released into the upper small intestine. Finally, the gallbladder releases bile to promote fat digestion. Assimilation of most nutrients occurs in the small intestine; the colon absorbs water, bile salts, and a few other substances to prepare the remainder of the colonic contents for elimination.

Regular elimination is also crucial to overall health and control of the level of toxicity in the body—constipation is actually a greater problem than most doctors and patients realize. Hydration, diet, level of physical activity, and stress all affect our eliminative function.

Health and proper functional integrity of the huge mucosal membrane surface area of the GI tract allow the proper assimilation of nutrients. Even minor disruptions related to inflammation or infection may cause abnormal absorption and increased barrier permeability. With increased intestinal permeability, absorption goes out of balance and larger-than-normal molecules get absorbed. This can cause allergic reactions and other abnormal immune responses. There is a delicate balance between the assimilation of needed nutrients and the exclusion of toxic substances. Abnormal organisms within the intestinal lumen may also produce toxins that can significantly affect mental and physical health. For example, an overgrowth of candida yeast may cause food fermentation and more biotoxins to be absorbed, which can affect energy, mood, and brain function. Also, certain pathogens within the GI tract may generate autoimmune reactions in the particularly vulnerable environment of the small bowel, where the majority of our immune cells are located.

Problems of dysbiosis, abnormal GI mucosal permeability, infection, and inflammation are exceedingly common and may cause both gastrointestinal complaints and other health concerns. This can be an important part of a health assessment. The GI tract is stressed and otherwise adversely affected by the following:

- Refined foods and sugar

- Excess fatty and rich foods

- Overeating and failing to chew more than once or twice per mouthful of food

- Drinking too much with meals, thus diluting our digestive juices and reducing our ability to properly break down food

- Lack of fiber and whole foods, specifically lacking fresh fruits, vegetables, whole grains, and legumes in the diet

- Eating too many different kinds of foods at a time and doing so over

the course of many years (one of the key causes of obesity and a chronic breakdown of digestive health and function)

- Food chemicals, pesticides, and environmental toxins

- Persistent use of alcohol, caffeine, and nicotine

- Use of prescription, over-the-counter, and recreational drugs

The GI tract is especially sensitive to emotional turmoil. A stressful lifestyle may adversely affect motility, digestive enzyme output, and overall function. More than thirty gut hormones have been identified, many of which also act as neurotransmitters. Chemical exposure (specifically ingested chemicals), travel, regular restaurant eating, and subsequent parasitic infections, or the overuse of antibiotics can cause intestinal dysfunction and disease. It may take years for the gut to recover from this kind of damage.

It is also important that the body maintain proper levels of friendly bacteria within the colon while their numbers remain low in concentration when progressing up the GI tract into the small intestine or stomach. Overgrowth of abnormal bacteria, fermenting yeasts, and parasites can disturb GI function, causing inflammation along the sensitive mucous membrane of the GI tract and thereby adversely affecting the assimilation of food and nutrients.

Abnormal permeability, often called *leaky gut*, creates GI imbalance, which can lead to systemic disease. Overconsumption of nonnutrient compounds and underconsumption or underassimilation of required nutrients may produce deficiencies and lead to allergies or other immune system problems. Inflammation or infection in the GI tract, food allergies, and the overuse of alcohol and non-steroid anti-inflammatory drugs (NSAIDs) can all cause problems with permeability. Disorders such as irritable bowel syndrome (IBS), colitis, Crohn's disease, rheumatoid arthritis, and HIV infections are frequently associated with leaky gut and permeability problems. A common condition involves fermentation from yeast overgrowth, specifically *Candida albicans* and other related candida species, which can lead to a large variety of symptoms and are often associated with permeability problems.

Of the trillions of microorganisms inhabiting the healthy GI tract, the friendly ones include the bacteria *Escherichia coli* (*E. coli*), various *Streptococci*, and *Lactobacillus acidophilus*, as well as *Lactobacillus bifidis* (*Bifidobacteria*), which is predominant in infants and children. However, many other undesirable organisms reside in the GI tract, particularly in the large intestine. These can include yeasts, abnormal bacteria such as *Klebsiella* (not always pathogenic) and *Citrobacter* species, a variety of pathogenic parasites, which include *Giardia lamblia* and *Blastocystis hominis*, and amoebas such as histolytica, hartmani, and coli.

HEALING THE GI TRACT

There are several ways to think about and approach healing the gastrointestinal tract. One of the most effective ways has been developed and taught by Jeff Bland, PhD, Leo Galland, MD, and others in their nutritional education seminars. This approach is an aspect of Functional (Physiological) Medicine. Preventive Medicine focuses on basic functions within the body, balancing or rebalancing them when they are not right through the use of supportive nutrients and appropriate natural substances, and of course, detoxification. This is similar to Orthomolecular Medicine, a concept coined by Linus Pauling and whose work and philosophy applying his truly biochemical term "Orthomolecular" (restoring health by supporting cellular health with the right nutrients in the right amounts) we continue through our medical group called Orthomolecular Health Medicine in San Francisco. We need to keep pursuing better ways to assess, heal, and support GI anatomy and physiology as a way to remedy illness and generate health.

There are many gastrointestinal tests that can be helpful in determining dysfunctions, diseases, and imbalanced microbes. These include basic X-rays and the scopes, such as gastroscopy (stomach from above), sigmoidoscopy, and colonoscopy (colon from below) as well as tests for digestive markers and all microbes, such as bacteria, yeasts, and parasites. These all allow for a deeper understanding of what might be causing gas and bloating, diarrhea and constipation, or abdominal pain. Gastroenterology specialists typically perform the scopes while more integrative practitioners perform some of these newer, functional tests through labs like Genova Diagnostics in North Carolina, Metametrix in Georgia, Doctor's Data, Inc. in Illinois, and Diagnos-Techs in Washington.

THE 5R GASTROINTESTINAL SUPPORT PLAN

The 5R is a progressive therapeutic program that normalizes the function, environment, and tissue health of the GI tract and must be tailored to the individual according to his or her particular evaluation. The 5R steps are the following:

1. **Rebalance—your diet, your lifestyle, and your life.** (This is a new "R" added to Dr. Jeffrey Bland's 4R Plan.) First, a healthy diet and lifestyle support a healthy digestive tract. Staying away from sugar, refined foods, and irritating substances such as caffeine and alcohol can make a big difference. Learning to deal with stress and developing coping and relaxation skills can help rebalance the GI tract's biochemistry and support better digestion and assimilation.

2. **Remove—any offending organisms and any food antigens,** particularly pathogenic microbes and/or foods that cause allergic and immunologic reactions. These include *Giardia lamblia*, abnormal types or levels of yeast organisms such as *Candida albicans*, and bacterial pathogens. Then, these can be treated with appropriate pharmaceutical or natural medications. I also encourage following an elimination diet that avoids allergenic, reactive foods and removes irritating substances such as caffeine, alcohol, refined sugar, and flour, and following a "hypoallergenic" diet that involves eliminating common food allergens such as cow's milk, eggs, gluten grains (wheat, rye, and barley), chocolate, coffee, and peanuts (and even soy products in some people). A diet of fruits, vegetables, rice and beans, some nuts and seeds, fish, and poultry is usually an improvement for most people, producing a reduction of symptoms and an increase in energy.

3. **Replace—inadequate amounts of hydrochloric acid (HCl), digestive enzymes, fiber, and pancreatic products.** Proper digestion reduces the allergenic and inflammatory effects that occur from malabsorption of larger, more complex molecules.

Replacement products are categorized as follows:

- Betaine and other forms of HCl

- Plant-derived digestive enzymes (proteases, amylases, lipases, and cellulases)

- Animal-derived enzymes (proteases, amylases, lipases, and elastases)

- Microbe-derived digestive enzymes

- Lactase enzyme supplements

- Fiber, both soluble and insoluble

4. **Reinoculate**—refers to the reintroduction or reflorastation of desirable bacterial flora as well as special nutrients such as fructooligosaccharides (FOS), which support the growth and function of friendly microorganisms. Reinoculation includes supplementation of symbiotic bacteria normally present in the healthy GI tract. These bacteria, called probiotics, include *Lactobacillus acidophilus* (also *bulgaricus* and *thermophilus*) and *Bifidobacterium bifidus* (also *longum, infantis*, and *breve*). There are many good products available in the marketplace. These probiotics are available primarily in powder form and as capsules or

Some Impressive GI Tract Facts

- The total GI mucosal surface is made up of many microscopic crypts and crevices, most of which are in the small intestine and have the interactive surface area equivalent to a tennis court.

- There are as many bacteria in a gram of stool as there are stars in the known universe.

- The microbes of the GI tract constitute a very metabolically active area of the body, second only to the liver.

- The total weight of the bacteria located in the colon of the average human equals approximately five pounds (or about the weight of our liver).

- The digestive organs manufacture nearly a gallon of juices per day to help digest and utilize the food we eat.

IMPORTANT ELEMENTS OF HEALTHY EATING

- **Eat whole foods,** especially fresh fruits, vegetables, whole grains, and vegetable proteins (beans, peas, lentils, nuts, and seeds).

- **We are what we eat.** Put only quality food into your body. Reduce refined foods, sugar, excess fatty and rich foods, and foods with additives or synthetic coloring. Avoid genetically engineered foods and those with chemical herbicides and pesticides by buying foods labeled organic.

- **Drink no more than 4 ounces of liquids with meals,** as it can dilute the digestive juices.

- **Drink 6 to 8 glasses of water daily,** plus herbal teas. Drink 2 to 3 glasses first in the morning and then 1 to 2 glasses an hour or so before lunch and dinner. **Liquid trace ionic minerals** help water move better into our cells and tissues.

- **Chew your food thoroughly,** eat in a relaxed environment, and relax yourself to prepare your body for nourishment.

- **Get sufficient fiber** in your diet by eating the majority of your foods from the first tip above and/or by taking additional psyllium seed husks, chia seeds, or flaxseed meal.

- **Use nutritional supplements** and herbs as appropriate. Supplement your digestive function as needed with hydrochloric acid, digestive enzymes, and pancreatic products.

- **Moderate your use of alcohol, caffeine, and nicotine.** Beware of excessive use of prescription, over-the-counter (OTC), and recreational drugs.

- **If you don't yet have an exercise program, set one up.** Do it regularly and with the right combination of activities that will provide strength, flexibility, endurance, and enjoyment.

- **Maintain regular elimination.** Your diet, exercise, and stress levels should allow your bowels to move at least once or twice daily. After illness or antibiotic use, replace friendly GI flora by taking probiotics (acidophilus and other positive digestive bacteria). If this is not sufficient to restore normal digestion and elimination, and your GI function stays irregular for more than a few weeks, seek the advice of a health-care practitioner.

tablets, although cultured yogurt or milk products also contain some Lactobacilli species.

5. **Repair—means providing nutritional support for the regeneration and healing** of the gastrointestinal lining and is probably the most important component of the 5R Program.

The GI mucosal cells represent the largest mass of biochemically active and proliferating cells in the body. Repair is needed when the structure or function of the gastrointestinal mucosa loses its integrity. Loss of integrity can result from infection (particularly from parasites or yeast), food allergy, chronic nutritional deficiency, chemical exposure, inflammatory bowel disease, and general dysbiosis (abnormal microbial balance).

Proper detoxification begins with understanding gastrointestinal function and its effect on overall health and will improve your health, vitality, and the functioning of your gastrointestinal tract. This, in turn, reduces the chance of degenerative and chronic diseases and helps slow the aging process. Remember, prevention is the key!

Some of the important nutrients for healing the GI tract include the amino acid L-glutamine, pantothenic acid, zinc, vitamin A, antioxidants (such as vitamins C and E, beta-carotene, and selenium), the bioflavonoid quercetin, essential fatty acids, inulin, and fiber (particularly the soluble kind). Herbs such as aloe vera, licorice root, and marshmallow root also have positive healing effects on the mucosal lining of the gastrointestinal tract. These nutrients play a key role in GI mucosal cell differentiation, growth, function, and repair. The sidebar on pages 38–39 describes these important nutrients.

NUTRIENTS FOR HEALING THE GI TRACT

For deeper discussions of these important nutrients, see my book, *Staying Healthy with Nutrition*.

1. **L-glutamine** is a nonessential amino acid used as fuel by active cells, particularly the enterocytes (mucosal lining cells) of the GI tract. Glutamine is also used directly as a fuel by brain cells and can help with control of alcohol and sugar cravings.

2. **Pantothenic acid** (vitamin B$_5$) is necessary for protein synthesis and energy production, both of which are involved in the tissue healing process.

3. **Ascorbic acid (vitamin C)** is essential for collagen formation, which is the basis for connective tissue repair, wound healing, and general tissue strength. It also works as an antioxidant to counter free radicals that can damage and inflame tissues.

4. **Vitamin A (retinol) and beta-carotene**, the nontoxic precursor of vitamin A, is needed for normal growth, function, and repair of epithelial cells, including those in the GI mucosa. Taking both nutrients ensures proper levels of vitamin A.

5. **Vitamin E** is an essential antioxidant that defends cell membrane integrity and function, thus helping to protect active enzyme systems within the cells.

6. **Zinc** (picolinate and citrate are a couple of bioavailable sources) is essential to tissue health and repair, enzyme function, the integrity of the cell membrane structure, and cell replication. Research from France indicates zinc can be unusually effective in healing GI tissue inflammation.

7. **Selenium** is an important antioxidant for chemical detoxification; it protects GI tract cells from damage and allows appropriate repair. This trace mineral is best taken as supplemental selenomethionine, which is absorbed better as bound to the amino acid.

8. **Quercetin** is a bioflavonoid with antihistamine and anti-inflammatory effects, useful in reducing food allergy reactions and helping in tissue repair.

9. **Essential fatty acids (EFAs)** help maintain the integrity of cell membranes and protect and heal the cells and tissues. Good sources include gamma linolenic acid (GLA) from evening primrose oil and borage oil, as well as eicosapentaenoic acid (EPA) and docosahexaenoic acid (DHA) from fish oils. Fresh organic flaxseed oil offers a good source of EFAs as well.

10. **Inulin** is a storage carbohydrate found in onions and Jerusalem artichokes (sunchokes) that acts as fuel for colon epithelial cells and promotes healing and energy generation.

11. **Aloe vera**, in its purified and extracted juice form, is both soothing and healing to the GI tract mucosa and tissue. Aloe vera capsules can also act as a laxative.

12. **Licorice root**, and specifically deglycyrrhized licorice (DGL), has an anti-inflammatory effect on the GI tract. DGL is particularly helpful in healing ulcers and other stomach inflammations.

13. **Marshmallow root** soothes and heals the gastrointestinal mucosa.

14. **Glutathione, L-cysteine, and N-acetylcysteine (NAC)** provide fuel and act as protective antioxidants and detoxification supporters for the GI mucosa and cellular enzyme systems.

15. **Fiber**, especially the soluble type, such as pectins and gels from fruits and vegetables, protects and promotes proper movement of feces through the GI tract without irritation. Insoluble fiber may also help lessen gut toxicity.

16. **Fructooligosaccharides (FOS)** fuels colon bacteria and protects colon cells from pathogenic infections. Some yeast and bacterial strains use FOS as a food source.

17. **Calories** from fresh fruits and vegetables, whole grains, seeds, and legumes are needed to repair damaged or inflamed tissues and maintain energy levels during the GI tract healing program.

18. **Probiotics** are essential as the healthy bacteria that support bowel function and protect us from bad bugs. They are especially needed to replenish the colon bacteria after taking antibiotics. There are many Lactobacilli organisms and Bifidobacteria, plus other special ones like *Saccharaomyces*.

CHAPTER FOUR

Fasting and Juice Cleansing

FASTING IS THE SINGLE GREATEST natural healing therapy I know. It is nature's ancient, universal remedy for many problems, used instinctively by animals when ill and by earlier cultures for healing and spiritual purification. When I first discovered fasting more than thirty-five years ago, I felt as if it had saved my life. My stagnant energies began flowing; my allergies, aches, and pains disappeared; and I became more creative and vitally alive. I still find fasting both a useful personal tool and an important therapy for many medical and life problems.

Most of the conditions for which fasting are appropriate result from excess food intake rather than from undernourishment. Dietary abuses generate many chronic degenerative diseases such as atherosclerosis, hypertension, heart disease, allergies, diabetes, cancer, and substance abuse, which undermine our health and precede the breakdown of the body. Fasting is not only therapeutic but, more important, acts in preventing many conditions. It often becomes the catalyst for shifting from unhealthy or abusive habits to a more healthful lifestyle in general.

As we use the term here, fasting refers to the avoidance of solid food and the intake of liquids only. True fasting would be the total avoidance of anything by mouth. (And I have recently heard from some people who do "dry fasting," which is nothing by mouth, well, except air of course. Truthfully, dry fasting sounds a bit crazy, extreme, and unhealthy to me because one of the keys to detoxifying is to have the fluids flush the toxins from the body.) The most stringent form of fasting allows drinking water exclusively; more liberal fasting includes the juices of fresh fruits and vegetables as well as herbal teas. All of these methods generate a high degree of detoxification—eliminating toxins from the body. Individual experiences with fasting depend upon the overall condition of the body, mind, and attitude. Detoxification can be intense and may either temporarily increase sickness or be immediately helpful and uplifting.

Juice fasting is commonly used as an effective cleansing plan. Fresh juices are easily assimilated and require minimal digestion, while still supplying many nutrients and stimulating our body to clear wastes. It is also safer than water fasting as juice supports the body nutritionally (at least somewhat) while cleansing and hence maintains energy levels, producing better detoxification and a quicker recovery.

I believe fasting is the "missing link" in the Western diet and lifestyle. Most people overeat, eat too often, and eat a high-protein, high-fat, acid-congesting diet more consistently than is necessary. If we regularly eat a balanced, well-combined, more alkalinizing diet high in fresh vegetables and fruits, we will have less need for fasting and toning plans (although both are still highly beneficial performed at intervals throughout the year).

Detoxification is a time when we allow our cells and organs to breathe and restore themselves. However, we do not necessarily need to fast to experience some cleansing. Even minor dietary shifts, including an increase in fluids, more raw foods, and fewer congesting foods, will initiate and promote better bodily function and improved detoxification. For example, a vegetarian or macrobiotic diet will be very cleansing and purifying to someone on a heavier diet. The general process of detoxification is discussed thoroughly in chapter 2. Here we focus on the history, benefits, and therapeutic use of fluid fasting.

Fasting is a time-proven remedy, with human origins going back many thousands of years. Voluntary abstinence from food has been a tradition in most religions and is still used as a spiritual purification rite. Religions such as Christianity, Judaism, Islam, Buddhism, and Hinduism have encouraged fasting as penance, preparation for ceremony, purification, mourning, sacrifice, divine union, and enhancement of mental and spiritual powers. The Bible is filled with stories of people fasting for purification and communion with God. The Essenes, authors of the *Dead Sea Scrolls*, also advocated fasting as one of their primary methods of healing and spiritual revelation, as described in *The Essene Gospel of Peace* (translated by Edmond Bordeaux Szekely from the third-century Aramaic manuscript).

Philosophers, scientists, and physicians across time have fasted as a means to promote life and recover health after sickness. Socrates, Plato, Aristotle, Galen,

Paracelsus, and Hippocrates all used fasting therapy. Many of today's spiritual teachers also recommend fasting as a useful tool. In a lecture titled "Healing by God's Unlimited Power" (1947), Paramahansa Yogananda suggested that fasting increased our natural resistance to disease, stating, "Fasting is a natural method of healing. When animals or savages are sick, they fast. Most diseases can be cured by judicious fasting. Unless one has a weak heart, regular short fasts have been recommended by the yogis as an excellent health measure."

Through the centuries, physicians and healers have treated a variety of maladies with fasting, acknowledging that ignorance of how to live in accordance with nature may be our greatest disease. Our inherent knowledge of how to live according to the natural laws and spiritual truths leads to the sacred wisdom of life and subsequent good health. Knowing when and how long to fast is part of this knowledge. Through fasting, we can turn our energies inward, where we can use them for healing, clarity, and change.

Physicians with a spiritual orientation tend to be more inclined than others to employ fasting, both personally and in their practices. Many of my own life transitions were stimulated and supported through fasting; when I have felt blocked or needed creative energy in my writing, fasting has been very useful. In *Spiritual Nutrition and the Rainbow Diet* (currently published as *Spiritual Nutrition*), physician and spiritual teacher Gabriel Cousens, MD, includes an excellent chapter on fasting in which he describes his theories and his own forty-day regime. According to Dr. Cousens,

> . . . *fasting in a larger context, means to abstain from that which is toxic to mind, body, and soul. A way to understand this is that fasting is the elimination of physical, emotional, and mental toxins from our organism, rather than simply cutting down on or stopping food intake. Fasting for spiritual purposes usually involves some degree of removal of oneself from worldly responsibilities. It can mean complete silence and social isolation during the fast which can be a great revival to those of us who have been putting our energy outward.*

From a medical point of view, fasting is not utilized often enough. We take vacations from work to relax, recharge, and gain new perspectives on our life—why not take occasional breaks from food? (Or, for that matter, from excessive television viewing or communication devices?) To break the habit of eating three meals a day is a challenge for most of us. When we stop and let our stomachs remain empty, our bodies go into an elimination cycle, and most people will experience some withdrawal symptoms, especially when toxicity exists. Symptoms include headaches, irritability, or fatigue. As with all allergies or addictions, eating again assuages these symptoms.

Fasting is a useful therapy for so many conditions and people. Those who tend to develop congestive symptoms do well with fasting; congestive acidic conditions include colds, flus, bronchitis, mucus congestion, and constipation (see the long list of symptoms and medical conditions that may benefit from detoxification on page 44). If not addressed, such conditions can lead to headaches, chronic intestinal problems, skin conditions, and more severe ailments. Most of us living in Western, industrialized nations suffer from both overnutrition and undernutrition.

We take in excessive amounts of foods containing potentially toxic nutrients, such as fats, sugars, and chemicals, and inadequate amounts of many essential vitamins and minerals, primarily contained in natural foods. The resulting congestive diseases are characterized by excess mucus and sluggish elimination; deficiency problems result from either poor nourishment or ineffective digestion and assimilation. Juice fasting supplies nutrients while still allowing for the elimination of toxins.

Juice fasting/cleansing can be used both to detoxify from drugs and when embarking on a new lifestyle transition, provided there are no contraindications (discussed later in this chapter). Short-term fasting is versatile and generally safe; however, when used to treat medical conditions, proper supervision should be employed. Many physicians, chiropractors, acupuncturists, and nutritionists feel comfortable overseeing people during cleansing/ detox programs, and I encourage you to

seek them out if your condition warrants supervision. Make sure they're not only theoretical but also practical in their own self-knowledge and experience. The following bullet points relate to the chart on page 44.

- The use of fasting as a treatment for **fevers** is controversial. It shouldn't be. Consuming liquids generates less heat, and this helps cool the body. With fever, we need more liquids than usual.

- Some cases of **fatigue** respond well to fasting, particularly when the fatigue results from congested organs and stalled energy. With fatigue that results from chronic infection, nutritional deficiency, or serious disease, added nourishment is probably called for as opposed to fasting.

- **Back pain** caused by muscular tightness and stress (rather than from bone disease or osteoporosis) is usually alleviated with a lighter diet or juice fasting. Much tightness and soreness along the back results from colon or other organ congestion; in my experience, poor bowel function and constipation are commonly associated with back pain. Fasting also helps reduce body inflammation, which is at the core of most pains.

- **Patients with mental illness,** ranging from anxiety to schizophrenia, may be helped by fasting.

Although this may sound sensational, the purpose of fasting in this case, however, is not to cure these problems, but rather to help understand the relationship of foods, chemicals, and drugs to mental and emotional functioning. Additional allergies and environmental reactions are not at all uncommon in people with mental illness. True, the release of toxins or lack of nourishment during fasting may worsen psychiatric problems; if, however, the patient is strong and congested, fasting may be helpful. The supervision of a health-care provider is important for patients with mental illness.

• People often attempt to remedy **obesity by fasting,** although that is not the best use of this healing technique. Fasting is actually too temporary an approach for overweight dieters and may even generate feasting reactions in people coming off the fast. A better solution would be a more gradual change of diet with a longer-term weight-reduction plan—something that will replace old dietary habits and food choices with new ones. However, a short five- to ten-day fast can motivate people to make the necessary dietary changes and renew commitments to proper eating. Some very obese patients who have needed to shed weights of a hundred pounds or more have been on month-long water fasts supervised in hospitals. Other patients have had their jaws wired shut, allowing them to ingest only fluids through straws. Still others have surgery to shrink their stomach size, and these stomach bypasses have become more popular in recent years. Newer fasting programs incorporate a variety of protein-rich powders for meals. These are also usually medically supervised and are for people who are at least thirty to fifty pounds overweight. These prepackaged, high-protein, low-calorie diets allow patients to burn more fat. Although these programs are not nearly as healthful as vital juice fasts, they are more nutritionally supportive over a longer period of time and can be used on an outpatient basis fairly safely if people are monitored regularly. In theory, they provide all the needed vitamins, minerals, and amino acids to sustain life while helping many people lower their weight, blood fats, blood pressure, and blood sugars. However, as with any weight-loss program, success depends upon participant motivation to change personal diets and habits permanently, as fluctuating weights may actually be more harmful than just remaining overweight.

- **Many obese people are also deficient in nutrients** because they eat a highly refined, fatty, sweet diet. They are often fatigued and need to be nourished first before they will do well on any fast. A well-balanced, low-calorie, low-chemical, high-nutrient diet with lots of exercise is still the best way to reduce and maintain a good weight and figure.

- **Fasting to treat cancer is a controversial topic** but is used by many alternative clinics outside the United States. Because of cancer's extremely debilitating effects, this may not be wise. Juice fasting may be helpful in the early stages of cancer and is definitely a preventive measure because it reduces toxicity. Anyone with cancer needs adequate nourishment; adding fresh juices to an already wholesome diet can promote mild detoxification and enhance overall vitality. Consult with an experienced practitioner first for individual treatment guidance.

THE PROCESS AND BENEFITS OF FASTING

Although the results of fasting will vary depending upon the individual condition of the faster, there are a number of metabolic changes and experiences common to all. First, fasting is a catalyst for change and an essential part of transformational medicine. It promotes relaxation, energizes the body, mind, and emotions, and supports a greater spiritual awareness. Many fasters let go of past experiences and develop a positive attitude toward the present. Having plenty of energy to get things done and cleaning up our personal and community environment are also common responses to the cleansing process. Fasting definitely improves motivation and stimulates

SOME BENEFITS OF FASTING

Purification
Rejuvenation
More energy
Rest for digestive organs
Greater abdominal peace
Clearer skin
Sense of personal beauty
Anti-aging effects
Improved senses (vision, hearing,
    taste)
Self-confidence
Reduction of allergies
Weight loss
Clothes fit more comfortably
Drug detoxification

Better resistance to disease
Spiritual awareness
More restful sleep
More relaxation
Greater motivation and optimism
New inspiration and creativity
More clarity, mental and emotional
Improved communications
Better organization
Cleaner personal space
Cleaner boundaries for energy use
Commitment to habit changes
Diet changes, long term

creative energy; it also enhances health, beauty, and vitality by letting many of the body systems rest.

Fasting is a multidimensional experience, affecting people physically, mentally, emotionally, and spiritually. Breaking down stored or circulating chemicals is its basic process; the blood and lymph also have the opportunity to be cleansed of toxins as their eliminative functions are reduced. Each cell has the opportunity to catch up on its work; with fewer new demands, cells can repair themselves and eliminate wastes. Most fasters experience a new vibrancy of their skin and clarity of mind and body. Most important, the liver can spend more time detoxifying the body and creating new

essential substances. Two to three quarts of water and juices daily (or even more for some people) are optimal during fasting to cleanse and support the body.

Metabolically, fasting initially reduces caloric intake to the point where the liver converts stored glycogen into glucose and energy. Body fat and fatty acids can be used for energy; however, the brain and central nervous system need direct glucose. With fasting, some protein breakdown occurs (less if calories are provided by juices). When glycogen stores are low, the body can convert protein into amino acids and energy—specifically the amino acids alanine and serine can be used to produce glucose. Fatty acids can also be a source of energy during fasting, as they convert into ketones (acetone bodies), which can be used by the body to prevent protein loss. With juice fasting, there is less ketosis (disrupted carbohydrate metabolism), and the simple carbohydrates provided by the juices are easily used for energy and cellular function. Liquid high-protein (fasting) diets and other weight-loss programs may burn more fat and generate more ketosis, but they also add more toxins and may create other health concerns.

Fasting increases the process of elimination and the release of toxins from the colon, kidneys, bladder, lungs, sinuses, and skin. This process can generate discharges such as mucus, which helps clear biochemical suffocation. Fasting helps us decrease this suffocation by allowing the cells to eliminate waste products, increase oxygenation, and improve cellular nutrition.

As for fasting symptoms, headache is not at all uncommon during the first day or two. Hunger is usually present for two or three days and then departs, leaving many people with a surprising feeling of deep "abdominal peace." When hungry, it is good to ask ourselves, "What are we hungry for?" Fasting is an excellent time to work on the psychological aspects of consumption. Fatigue or irritability may arise at times, as may dizziness or lightheadedness. Sensitivity is usually increased, and common sounds like the telephone, television, music, or the hum of a refrigerator or air conditioner may be more irritating. Our sense of smell is also exaggerated. Most people's tongues will develop a thick white or yellow fur coating, which can be scraped or brushed off. Bad breath and displeasing tastes in the mouth, or foul-smelling urine or stools, may occur.

Skin odor or skin eruptions such as small spots or painful boils may also appear, depending on the level of toxicity. Digestive upset, mucus-containing stools, flatulence, or even nausea and vomiting may also occur. Some people experience insomnia or bad dreams as their body releases poisons during the night. Wild dreams about weird foods are not uncommon. Believe me, the ultimate benefits are well worth the transient discomforts.

The mind may put up resistance, sending messages of doubt or fear that fasting is not right. This can be exaggerated by listening to other people's fears about your fasting. (If you are looking for excuses to not fast, they are everywhere.) Most symptoms will occur early on (if at all) and will pass. Generally, energy levels are good, although energy may go down every two or three days as the body excretes more wastes. It is at these times that resistance and fears (as well as new symptoms) may arise; if symptoms occur, it is wise to drink more fluids. However, most people will feel cleaner, better, lighter, more open, and more alive most of the time.

Old symptoms or patterns from the past may arise during fasts—again usually transiently—or new symptoms of detoxification may appear. Problems, often called "healing crises," that can occur with periodic cleansing are not usually predictable and can raise doubts and questions—is this a new problem or part of the healing process? Generally, time over a day or two will sort things out. We should use Hering's Law of Cure to guide us in making these judgment calls. It states that healing happens from the inside out, the top down, from more important (deeper, solid) organs like the kidneys and liver to less important ones, and from the most recent to the oldest symptoms. Most healing crises pass within a day or two, although some cleansers experience several days of cold symptoms or sinus congestion. If any symptom lasts longer than two or three days, it should be considered a side effect or new problem and should be addressed accordingly. If a problem worsens or causes concern (such as fainting, heart arrhythmias, or bleeding), the fast should be stopped and a doctor consulted.

CASE STUDY: K.F., AGE 38, MOTHER

I have been a patient of Dr. Haas for many years. He does inspire me to care for myself and my family as well as treat any problems that come up. I know he is always thinking of the safest and most natural way to treat us.

Therefore, when he told me about his detox groups, I elected to participate. I will briefly explain my experiences. I am basically healthy and not really overweight. Yet, I have had knee pains and some arthritis patterns since I was a teenager. And my energy does wax and wane over the month and year. I just couldn't figure out any of the causes.

First I did the Three-Week Autumn Detox Program with a large group of people. I got off sugar and caffeine, and then in the second week, off wheat, dairy, eggs, and the rest of the Sensitive Seven (sugar, corn, soy, and peanuts). Then, the third week, we started to bring some of these foods back. It was great! Immediately I could tell that wheat and dairy products made me sluggish and congested in my nose and head. And my knees felt better at first, and then the aches and pains came back. I didn't really connect with this because I had no thought that my twenty years of pain would have any relevance to this process. But, I did feel better overall.

In spring, Dr. Haas motivated me to do his ten-day Spring Cleanse (Juice Cleanse Diet), more of a juice diet. I was open, even though I was concerned about losing weight. However, I did make it through with the other twenty-five people. I felt amazing! And what's more, my knees were totally pain-free for the first time. Then, Dr. Haas encouraged me to come back into my diet slowly, which I was happy to do because I felt so good drinking juices and now eating lightly, mostly fresh fruits and vegetables. As I progressed into other foods, I saw that wheat, dairy, sugar, and corn syrup made my knees ache. It was very cool to connect this and gain power over this chronic pain. I say that because more than a year later, my knees and my body still feel much better. I would never have thought these simple food reactions could be contributing to this chronic problem. Thank you, Dr. Haas, for this experiential and awakening education.

Medical supervision is important for anyone in poor health or without fasting experience. If the fast is extended for more than three or four days, regular monitoring, including physical examinations and blood work, should be done weekly (particularly if there is any cause for concern). Fasting may not only reduce blood protein levels, but it will definitely lower blood fats. Uric acid levels may rise due to protein breakdown, while levels of some minerals such as potassium, sodium, calcium, or magnesium may drop. Iron levels are usually lower, and the red blood cell count may also drop slightly during this time. Lowered mineral levels can result in fatigue or muscle cramps; if these should occur, additional minerals (particularly calcium, magnesium, and potassium) should be taken, ideally in a powdered form for easy assimilation.

Nutritionally, fasting helps us appreciate the more subtle aspects of our diet, as less food and simple flavors will become more satisfying (even food aromas can be fulfilling). Mentally, fasting improves clarity and attentiveness; emotionally, it may make us more sensitive and aware of our feelings. Individuals may gain the clarity to make important decisions during this therapy. Fasting definitely supports the transformational, evolutionary process. Juice fasting offers a lesson in self-restraint and control of passions. This new and empowering sense of self-discipline can be highly motivating. Fasters who were once spectators suddenly become participants.

HAZARDS OF FASTING

If fasting is overused, it may create depletion and weakness in the body, lowering resistance and increasing susceptibility to disease. While fasting does allow the organs, tissues, and cells to rest and handle excesses, the body needs the nourishment provided by food to function after it has used up its stores.

Malnourished people should definitely not fast, nor should some overweight people who are undernourished. Others who should not fast include people with fatigue resulting from nutrient deficiency, those with chronic degenerative disease of the muscles or bones, and those who are underweight. Diseases associated with clogged or toxic organs respond better to fasting. Sluggish individuals who retain water or whose weight is concentrated in their hips and legs often do worse. Those with low daytime energy and more vitality at night (more yin or alkaline types) may not enjoy fasting either.

Fasting is not recommended for pregnant or lactating women, or for people who have weak hearts or weakened immunity. (However, most women can benefit from short juice cleanses during their menstrual cycle to help ease pain and other symptoms.) As I've previously mentioned, before or after surgery is not a good time to fast, as the body needs its nourishment to handle the stress and healing demands of the operation and to support tissue repair. Although some nutritional therapies for cancer include medically supervised fasting, I do not usually recommend fasting for cancer patients, particularly those with advanced problems. Ulcer disease is not something for which fasting is suggested, either, although fasting may be beneficial for other conditions present in a patient whose ulcer is under control.

Some clinics and fasting practitioners do believe in fasting for ulcers. In the first test case of the Master Cleanser, Stanley Burroughs claims to have cured a patient with an intractable ulcer. The two main ingredients of the Master Cleanser, citrus juice and cayenne pepper, are substances all the physicians had suggested this patient avoid; Dr. Burroughs deduced they might be the only things left to heal the ulcer, and perhaps he is right. I have certainly seen Master Cleanser do a lot of healing. The fasting process itself is helpful for ulcers as it reduces stomach acid and aids in tissue healing. Cayenne pepper, although hot, heals mucous membranes and is commonly recommended for ulcers in herbal medicines. So, even though peptic ulcers are on the contraindication list, some sufferers may be helped by fasting, especially with cabbage or vegetable juices.

As with any therapy, fasting has some potential hazards. Clearly, excessive weight loss and nutritional deficiencies may occur—a response more marked with longer water fasts and less likely with juices as they provide some calories and nutrients. Weakness may occur, or muscle cramps may result from mineral deficits. Sodium, potassium, calcium, magnesium,

---

CONTRAINDICATIONS FOR FASTING

- Underweight
- Fatigue
- Low immunity
- Weak heart
- Low blood pressure
- Cardiac arrhythmias
- Cold weather
- Pregnancy
- Nursing
- Pre- and post-surgery
- Cancer
- Peptic ulcers
- Nutritional deficiencies
- Children

---

and phosphorus losses occur initially but diminish after a week. Blood pressure drops, and this can lead to dizziness (especially when changing position from lying to sitting or from sitting to standing). Uric acid levels may rise without adequate fluid intake, although this is rare; high uric acid levels can cause some joint pains, as with a sore gouty toe.

Some research reports hormone levels change while fasting. Initially, the level of thyroid hormone falls, but it rises again in association with protein-sparing ketosis. Female hormone levels fall, possibly as a result of protein malnutrition, and this can lead to a lessening or loss of menstrual flow. Cessation of periods in women is also seen in longtime vegetarians (particularly those who exercise extensively), arising typically from nutrient depletion. Menstruation will usually rebalance with proper diet and nourishment.

Cardiac problems such as arrhythmias can occur with prolonged fasting, especially when there are preexisting problems. Extra beats, both ventricular and atrial, have been seen, and there have even been deaths from serious ventricular arrhythmias (the latter of which occur most often during long water fasts). Similar problems have turned up in people using any nutrient-deficient protein powders as a weight loss tool without supervision. All of these risks are minimized with juice fasts of no more than two week's duration or when basic minerals (potassium, calcium, and magnesium) are supplemented during water fasts. Having our progress monitored through physical exams, blood tests, and even electrocardiograms is another way to protect ourselves from the potential hazards of fasting.

Another side effect (really a side benefit) of fasting is the way it affects and changes our personal lives. Often we resist inner guidance, feelings, and desires to do something new or get out of a bad situation, but fasting brings these to the fore. Divorce, job changes, and residential moves are all more likely after fasts, as they stimulate self-realization, enhance our potential, and help us focus on the future. Also, when we feel better, some things that appear to be too challenging become more manageable and desirable. During fasting, many people have new sensitivity and renewed awareness of their job, mate, and home. It does help when couples do programs together. It is good to remember that fasting can be a catalyst for change, and this creates an extra stress during detoxification. However, when we can relax and observe what's going on, it helps create better understanding. Even though these insights and changes may be traumatic initially, I believe they are ultimately positive and help us follow our true nature.

HOW TO FAST

The general plan for fasting is best when it takes progressive steps. This is my adaptive, moderate approach for new fasters and unhealthy patients, leading to a stricter program for the more experienced. It is important to build slowly and take time to transition. Although many people do fine even when making extreme changes, such abruptness clearly maximizes the risks of fasting.

A sensible daily plan mixes fasting with eating. Each day can include a twelve- to fourteen-hour period of fasting from early evening through the night, as indeed breakfast was given that name to denote the time where we "break the fast" of the night. Many people eat very lightly or not at all in the early morning in order to extend their daily fast; this is more important if dinner or snacking extends into the later evening. However, if dinner is at an early time, a good breakfast can be consumed after water intake and some stretching and exercise.

In preparation for our first day of fasting, we may want to take some time (a few days to a week) to eliminate unhealthy foods or habits from our diet. Abstaining from alcohol, nicotine, caffeine, and sugar is very helpful before fasting. Red meats and other animal foods, including milk products and eggs, as well as wheat and baked goods could be avoided for a day or two before fasting, thus easing the transition. Intake of most nutritional supplements should also be curtailed as these are usually not recommended during a fast. Many people prepare for their fasts by consuming only fruit and vegetable foods for three or four days. These slowly detoxify the body so that the actual fast will be less intense.

The first one-day fast gives us a chance to see what a short fast can be like. Most of us find it is not so very difficult and does not cause major distress. Food is abstained from for thirty-six hours, from 8 p.m. one night until 8 a.m. two days later. Most people will feel a little hungry and may experience a few mild symptoms such as a headache or irritability by the end of the fasting day, usually around dinnertime. The first two days are generally challenging for everyone; feeling great usually begins around day three. So take a walk, take a nap, cut your nails, breathe, read a book, pray, and bathe instead of eating.

One of the ironies of fasting is that it can be the most difficult for those who need it the most; in these cases, people must start with the subtle diet changes discussed above. One transition protocol is the one-meal-a-day plan. The meal is usually eaten around 3 p.m.; water, juices, teas, and some fresh fruit or vegetable snacks can be eaten at other times. It is important the wholesome meal be neither excessive nor rich. Start with a protein and vegetable meal, such as fish and salad or steamed vegetables, or a starch and vegetable meal, such as brown rice and mixed steamed greens, carrots, celery, and zucchini. People on this plan detoxify slowly, lose some weight, and after a few days feel pretty sound. The chance of any strong symptoms developing during this transition time or during a subsequent fast is greatly minimized.

The next goal for those who have done a one-meal-a-day program is a one-day fast. The fasting then progresses to two- and three-day fasts with one or two days between them when light foods and more raw fruits and vegetables are consumed. This allows us to build up to longer lasting five- to ten-day fasts. When the transition is made slowly, even water fasting can be less intense (although I usually recommend juice fasts).

To avoid being excessively impatient, we need to make and adhere to a plan. It is important to continually observe and listen to your body and even keep notes in a journal. Get to know yourself and your nature. Once we have fasted successfully, we can continue to do one-day fasts weekly or a three-day fast every month if we need them. This experience helps us reconnect with ourselves and work toward a goal of optimum health. Meditation, exercise, fresh air and sunshine, massages, and baths are all essential and nourishing during this and any cleansing period.

WHEN TO FAST

The two key times for natural cleansing are the transitions from winter into spring and summer into autumn. In Chinese medicine, the transition times between seasons last about ten days before and after each equinox or solstice. For spring, this period runs from about March 10 through April 1; for autumn, it is from about September 11 through October 2. In cooler climates, where spring weather begins later and autumn weather earlier, the fasting could be scheduled appropriately. It is easier to do a natural cleansing when it is warm, as the body tends to cool down during fasting.

Master Cleanser

SERVES 1

> 2 tablespoons freshly squeezed lemon
>   or lime juice
> 1 tablespoon pure maple syrup (up to
>   2 tablespoons if you want to drop
>   less weight)
> Small pinch (¹/₁₀ teaspoon) of cayenne pepper
> 8 ounces filtered or spring water

Mix and drink 8 to 12 glasses throughout the day. Eat or drink nothing else except water, laxative herb tea, and peppermint or chamomile tea. Keep the mixture in a glass container (not plastic) or make it fresh each time. Rinse your mouth with water after each glass to prevent the lemon juice from hurting the enamel of your teeth. *Note:* You can make some of the concentrate in the morning and take it with you to work in a small plastic jar; add 8 ounces of water to about 3 tablespoons of the concentrate just before drinking. If you add the water to a whole quart or half gallon, the mixture gets extremely hot (spicy) when the cayenne disperses more in the water.

Furthermore, I encourage you to drink it by the glass rather than sip every few minutes. This method protects the teeth and allows the body not to overly respond to repetitive sugar/ carbohydrate absorption. We want a glass or two to act like a meal.

For a spring fast, I usually suggest lemon and/or greens as the focus of the cleansing. Diluted lemon water, lemon, and honey, or, my favorite, the Master Cleanser (see left), can be used.

Fresh fruit or vegetable juices diluted with equal amounts of water will also stimulate cleansing. Some good vegetable choices are carrots, celery, beets, and greens, such as spinach, chard, and kale. Soup broths can also be used. Juices with blue-green algae, spirulina, or chlorella provide more energy, as they contain quality protein (amino acids) and are easily assimilated.

Fasting can also be done in other seasons. Summer, with the warm weather, is a good time to fast for seven to ten days. Winter cleansing can be one day per month or longer, but warming diets, such as brown rice, vegetables, and miso soup can also be helpful. This can be done for two to three weeks. In autumn, a fast of at least three to five days can be done, using either water or a variety of juices. Juices could include the Master Cleanser, apple and/or freshly made grape juice (usually mixed with a little lemon and water to reduce sweetness), vegetable juices, and warm broths.

Autumn Rejuvenation Ration

From Bethany Argisle
SERVES 2

> 3 cups spring water
> 1 tablespoon chopped gingerroot
> 1 to 2 tablespoons miso paste
> 1 to 2 stalks green onion, chopped
> Chopped cilantro, to taste
> 1 to 2 pinches cayenne pepper
> 2 teaspoons extra virgin olive oil
> Juice of $1/2$ lemon

Bring the water to a boil, add the gingerroot, and simmer for 10 minutes. Stir in the miso paste to taste (do not allow the paste to boil). Turn off the heat. Then add the green onion, cilantro, cayenne, olive oil, and lemon juice. Remove from the stove, cover, and steep for 10 minutes.

HOW LONG TO FAST

We can either follow a specific time schedule or listen closely to our own individual cycles and needs. Paying attention to your energy level and degree of congestion, and observing the tongue and its coating, will offer helpful cleansing guidelines. As we gain some fasting experience, we will become more attuned to specific times when we need to strengthen or lighten our diets and when we need to cleanse. If we are under stress, have been overindulging, or have developed some congestive symptoms, we need to lighten our diets and possibly cleanse. The odor of our urine, breath, and sweat are tell-tale signs of cleansing in action.

Breaking a Fast

Ending or stopping a fast and beginning to eat again also take some monitoring. Things to watch include energy level, weight, detoxification symptoms, tongue coating, and degree of hunger. If our energy falls for more than a day or if our weight gets too low, we should come off the fast. If symptoms are particularly intense or sudden, it is possible we need food. Generally, the tongue is a good indicator of our state of toxicity or clarity.

With fasting, the tongue usually becomes coated with a white, yellow, or gray film. This signals the body's cleansing process, and it will usually clear when the detox cycle is complete. However, tongue observation is not a foolproof indicator. Some people's tongues are coated very little, while others will remain coated even after cleansing. If in doubt, it is better to make the transition back to food and then cleanse again later. Hunger is another sign of readiness to move back into eating, as it is often minimal during cleansing times. Occasionally, people are very hungry throughout a fast, but most lose interest in food from day three to seven and then experience real, deep-seated hunger once again. This is a sign to begin eating, carefully.

Breaking a fast must be well planned and executed slowly and carefully to prevent the creation of symptoms and sickness. It is suggested we take half of our total cleansing time to move back into our regular diet, which is hopefully now better planned and more healthful. Our digestion has been at rest, so we need to chew our foods very well. If we have fasted on water alone, we need to prepare our digestive tract with diluted juices, perhaps beginning with a few teaspoons of fresh orange juice in a glass of water and progressing to stronger mixtures throughout the day. Diluted fresh grape or orange juice will stimulate the digestion.

Arnold Ehret, a European fasting expert and proponent of the mucusless diet, suggests fruits and fruit juices should not be used right after a meat eater's first fast because they may coagulate intestinal mucus and cause problems. A meat eater's colon bacteria are probably different from a vegetarian's. Consequently, fruit sugars like those in the juices may not be tolerated well; instead, the active gram-positive anaerobic bacteria in the meat eater will produce more toxins. Extra acidophilus supplements continued on a regular basis help shift colon ecology in meat eaters and can even be used during cleanses.

With juice fasting, it is easier to transition back to food. A raw or cooked low-starch vegetable, such as spinach or other greens, is quite appropriate. A little sauerkraut also helps stimulate the digestive function. A laxative-type meal including grapes, cherries, or soaked or stewed prunes can also be used to initiate eating, as they keep the bowels moving. Some experts say the bowels should move within an hour or two after the first meal and, if not, an enema should be used. Some people do a saltwater flush before their first day of food by drinking a quart of water containing 2 teaspoons of dissolved sea salt. Be careful. (See more on colon cleansing on page 75.) Our individual transit times vary in response to laxatives and saltwater.

However you make the transition, go slowly, chew well, and do not overeat or mix too many foods at any meal. Start with simple vegetable meals as described above. Fruit should be eaten alone. By the second day, well-cooked, watery brown rice or millet is handled well by most people. From there, progress slowly through grains and vegetables. Some nuts, seeds, or legumes can be added, and then richer protein foods, if these are desired. Returning to food is a crucial time for learning individual responses or reactions. Self-observation gives us an opportunity to

OTHER ASPECTS OF HEALTHY FASTING

- **Fresh air:** vital for oxygenation of the body's cells and tissues.

- **Sunshine:** source of vitamin D, but avoid excessive exposure.

- **Water:** bathing is very important to cleanse the skin.

- **Steams and saunas:** support detoxification.

- **Skin brushing:** using a dry, soft brush prior to bathing stimulates the skin.

- **Exercise:** both relaxing and energizing, exercise aids in eliminating wastes and thus helps preventing toxicity symptoms. Walking, bicycling, and swimming, as examples, can be done during a fast, although activities that are risky or dangerous should be avoided.

- **No drugs:** neither over-the-counter nor recreational drugs should be used during a fast; only mandatory prescription medications are acceptable. Avoiding alcohol, nicotine, and caffeine is imperative.

- **Vitamin supplements:** these are not used during fasting, and thus no program of nutrients will follow at the end of this chapter. Supplemental fiber, such as psyllium husks, can help detoxify the colon. Special chlorophyll foods such as green barley, chlorella, spirulina, or blue-green algae may enhance vitality and purification. Occasionally, some mineral support (especially potassium, calcium, magnesium) with vitamin C in powdered or liquid form helps prevent cramps or adds support during an extended fast. Some people even use amino acids or other vitamin powders. These supplemental nutrients are really best used when consumed with foods. (See chapter 6 for more on supplements and detoxification.)

- **Colon cleansing:** an essential part of healthy fasting. Some form of bowel stimulation is recommended. Colonic irrigations with water performed by a trained therapist (colon hydrotherapist) with modern equipment are the most thorough. These can be done at the beginning, midpoint, and end of the fast. It is suggested enemas be used at least every other day, especially if they are the primary cleansing method. Fasting clinics often suggest enemas be used daily or several times a day. With these, water alone is used to flush the colon of toxins. It may be helpful for an enema or a laxative preparation to be used the day before the fast begins, to lessen initial toxicity. Herbal laxatives are commonly taken orally during fasting, and many formulas are available either as capsules or for making tea. These include cascara sagrada, senna leaves, licorice root, buckthorn, rhubarb root, aloe vera, and prepared formulas. The saltwater flush (drinking a quart of warm water with 2 teaspoons of dissolved sea salt) can be used first thing in the morning or on alternate days throughout the fast to flush the entire intestinal tract, although it is not recommended for those with hypertension or who are salt-sensitive or retaining water.

- **Work and creativity:** staying busy helps break our cravings for food. Most fasters experience a boost in energy and expanded creativity and, naturally, find lots to do.

- **Clean up:** not only your body but also your environment. Make a clean sweep of your home and workplace, including your desk, office, closets, cupboards, car, garage, attic, and basement. If you want to prepare for the new, you will need to clear out the old.

- **Fast with others:** fasting with a group can generate strong emotional bonds and provide invaluable additional support. Fasters often report feeling more spiritually attuned, and for many, it is helpful to have others with whom to share this. Call our clinic or another that offers this service.

- **Embrace the naysayers:** not everyone will understand or endorse what you're doing—but instead of avoiding them or dismissing their opinions, be grateful for their care and concern. Share your knowledge, explain the goals of your program, and ask for their support. You may be pleasantly surprised.

- **Economic benefits:** you'll save time, money, and a fortune in future health-care costs. Many of us will be inspired to share more of ourselves when we are freed from food.

- **Meditation and relaxation:** important aspects of fasting that help clear stresses and bring us back in touch with our innermost selves.

- **Spiritual practice and prayer:** fasting can be an effective catalyst, providing us with inner fuel to live with purpose and passion.

see destructive dietary habits and discover specific food intolerances. You may wish to keep notes at this time. If you respond poorly to a food, avoid it for a week or so, and then eat it alone to see how it feels. This is when food allergies may be revealed.

JUICE SPECIFICS

Some juices work better for certain people or conditions. In general, diluted fresh juices of raw organic fruits and vegetables are best. Canned and frozen juices should be avoided. Some bottled juice may be used, but fresh squeezed or extracted is best, as long as it is used soon after processing. Lemon juice, wheatgrass, or a little ginger or garlic juice can be added to drinks for vitality and to stimulate cleansing.

Water and other liquids increase waste elimination. Lemon tends to loosen and draw out mucus and is especially useful for liver cleansing. Diluted lemon juice with or without a little honey or the Master Cleanser (page 53) loosens mucus quickly, so if this is used we need to cleanse the bowels regularly to prevent getting sick. Most vegetable juices are milder than lemon juice.

Each juice contains nutritional compounds and physiological actions found to prevent and support the healing of specific health conditions. Fresh juices are like natural vitamin pills with a very high assimilation rate that do not require the work of digestion.

The juices of apples, grapes, oranges, and carrots are good cleansing juices but might be minimized for weight loss because they are high in calories. Juices more helpful for weight loss include grapefruit, lemon, cucumber, and greens such as lettuce, spinach, or parsley. Also, a variety of juices can be used in a fast, prepared fresh daily. Keep recipes of your favorite new combinations.

To prepare juices, we want to start with the freshest and most chemical-free fruits and vegetables possible. They should be cleaned or soaked and stored properly. If not organic, they should be peeled, especially if they are waxed. With root vegetables such as carrots or beets, the above-ground ends should be trimmed. Some people drop their vegetables into a pot of boiling water for a minute or so to clean them before juicing. Use organic produce to avoid chemical herbicides and pesticides.

The right juicer is important. **Citrus juicers** are the simplest type of juicers. There are a number of handheld citrus juicers. For example, OXO makes a variety of efficient, handheld citrus juicers. **Motorized citrus juicers** basically press and squeeze the juice from the rind of a cut piece of fruit. They are very simple, easy to clean, and inexpensive. **Centrifugal juice extractors** have powerful high-speed motors that spin the produce to extract the juice. They are fast and the cheapest of the various electric juicers. **Masticating juice extractors** have blades that break up the produce. They run at a lower speed so they don't get as hot as the centrifugal juicers. This is a more healthful way to make juice, because heat can destroy enzymes and antioxidants in the juice. **Triturating juice extractors** work the same as masticating juice extractors except that they have two gears that run extremely close to each other and are very effective at extracting as much juice as possible. They are exceptionally good for wheatgrass and leafy greens. They are also the most expensive and require a little more time to clean. Blenders are not really juicers (what they produce is more like liquid salad) but can be used to puree soups or make smoothies. These drinks can also be used for a fast because they are high in fiber and nutrients. I once did an energizing week-long fast with two blender drinks a day—fruits in the morning and vegetables in the late afternoon—with teas and water in between.

CONCLUSION

When we overdo it with food or other substances, we need to return to the cycle of a daily night fast of twelve to fourteen hours and eating one main meal and two lighter ones. For low-weight, high-metabolism people, two larger or three moderately sized meals are probably needed. If we eat a heavier evening meal, we may need only a light breakfast, and vice versa. Through awareness and experience, we can find our individual nutritional needs and fulfill them with ease.

Fasting can easily become both a way of life and an effective dietary practice. Over a period of time we can go from symptom cleansing to preventive fasting. We should support ourselves regularly with a balanced, wholesome diet, and fast at specific times to treat symptoms and/or to enhance our vitality and spiritual practice. If we could devote one day per week to purification and a cleansing diet, the path of health would be smooth indeed.

Choosing healthy foods, chewing well, and maintaining good colon function all minimize our need for fasting. However, if we do get out of balance, we can employ one of the oldest treatments known to humans, the instinctive therapy for many illnesses, nature's doctor, therapist, and tool for preventing disease—FASTING!

JUICES AND THE CONDITIONS AND/OR ORGANS THEY MAY PREVENT AND/OR HELP HEAL

Note: The information in this chart has been developed from our clinical experience as well as some 75 studies on the benefits of fruit and vegetable juices on various health and disease conditions. For readers interested in pursuing more in-depth research, there are many published studies via pubmed.gov, which is a free resource from the US National Library of Medicine and the National Institutes of Health. The Center for Disease Control (CDC) provides a helpful list of nutrients from fruit and vegetable sources at www.fruitsandveggiesmatter.gov/benefits/index.html.

- **Apple**—heart disease, colon polyps and cancer, lymphoma, diabetes, Parkinson's, lung cancer, melanoma

- **Beet greens**—breast cancer, melanoma and diabetes, liver and gallbladder support, bone health

- **Beets**—blood and liver support, joints

- **Black cherry**—colon support, gout, menstruation

- **Broccoli**—gallbladder health, arthritis pain, heart health, lung cancer, prostate health, melanoma, bladder cancer

- **Cabbage**—high cholesterol, ulcers, Parkinson's, colon cancer and colitis, prostate cancer, melanoma

- **Carrots**—eye health and vision, lung and colon cancer, memory, non-Hodgkin's lymphoma, heart disease, melanoma

- **Celery**—kidneys and breast cancer, weight issues

- **Cherries** (tart)—toxic exposure, insomnia

- **Citrus**—high cholesterol, endometrial cancer, diabetes, vascular health, non-Hodgkin's lymphoma, melanoma

- **Collard greens**—breast cancer, memory, high cholesterol

- **Cucumber**—swelling, blood sugar balance

- **Garlic**—colds and flu, heart and vascular health, Parkinson's disease, many cancers

- **Grapes**—cardiovascular disease, melanoma, inflammation, arthritis

- **Kiwi**—cancer, arthritis, inflammation, colds

- **Leafy greens**—heart health, breast cancer, high cholesterol, diabetes, prostate cancer, colon cancer, melanoma

- **Lemons**—cholesterol, liver support, allergies and asthma, colds, weight management

- **Mustard greens**—high cholesterol

- **Papaya**—heart health, digestion, human papilloma viral infections, melanoma

- **Parsley**—kidney health, edema, inflammation, osteoarthritis, breast cancer

- **Pear**—stomach and lung cancer, gallbladder, macular degeneration, Alzheimer's disease

- **Peas**—stomach, indigestion, hemorrhoids, colitis

- **Pineapple**—allergies, arthritis, digestion, inflammation, edema, hemorrhoids

- **Potatoes**—macular degeneration, breast cancer, Alzheimer's disease

- **Radishes**—weight management, cholesterol

- **Spinach**—heart health, vision, blood support, bone density, enlarged prostate, macular degeneration, esophageal and colon cancer, headaches, cataracts, diabetes, non-Hodgkin's lymphoma, Parkinson's, breast cancer, diabetes

- **Watercress**—prostate cancer, edema, toxin removal

- **Watermelon**—kidneys, swelling, arthritis, lung cancer, breast cancer, prostate cancer, melanoma

- **Wheatgrass**—detox, liver and blood support, intestines

CHAPTER FIVE

The Detox Diet and Other Purifying Diets

BEFORE WE APPROACH THE DETOX DIET, we first want to give you some preventive medicine guidelines to follow so you won't need to detoxify as often. Instead, learn to eat and live in a way that creates and supports health, vitality, and longevity. The first step is to follow a nontoxic diet (see page 64). If we do this regularly, we have less need for cleansing. If we have not been eating this way, we should detoxify first and then make these more permanent changes. And of course, as we exercise and stretch regularly, rest and sleep well, and take a great attitude toward life and others, this all will keep our stress low and our health high.

I mention avoiding gluten as part of a healthy diet. Although this is not essential for everyone, it does help many people feel better with better energy, thinking, and digestion. Gluten is a protein joined with starch that is allergenic for many, and it is contained in wheat products, rye, and barley. There is also some in spelt and triticale. Oats and corn are less reactive typically, and buckwheat and quinoa are often well handled. Overall, following elimination diets is a way to sort out what works and what does not for each individual.

Another aspect of the nontoxic diet is avoiding drugs (over-the-counter, prescription, and recreational) and substituting natural remedies such as nutritional supplements, herbs, and homeopathic medicines, all of which have fewer side effects. I often do this first, before suggesting or taking prescription drugs.

Feeling Good as We Age

Most of us want to be healthy and not get old. Well, we are all going to become older in years at least; yet, the key is not to feel too old. In the modern world that's simply not the case. Due to our diets and lifestyle (and living longer, of course), many feel old and ill too early in life. We can change that for the better. I believe that's the case with me. I really believe my nearly forty years of detoxification practice and yearly cleanses have helped me look and feel youthful and at least delay the aging problems most of my family and relatives have experienced with diseases, doctors, and drugs due to hypertension, diabetes, and high cholesterol. In my mid-sixties now, I have no diagnoses, doctors, or drugs and feel good most every day. I want that for you too, and of course, the earlier you start with excellent self-care, the more likely that will be. Stay healthy! That's the key.

Other natural therapies, such as acupuncture, massage, osteopathic, and chiropractic care may help in treating certain problems so that we will not need drugs for them. Avoiding or minimizing exposure to chemicals at home and at work is also important. One way we can do this is by substituting chemically based personal products with natural cleansers, cosmetics, and clothing.

THE DETOX DIET

One of my favorite cleansing/detox programs is the Detox Diet. It is a simple eating program I have used with many thousands of people. I find it to be a great catalyst for healing—providing more energy, fewer debilitating symptoms (such as aches and pains or congestion and allergies), and the inspiration necessary for making permanent changes in diet and lifestyle habits.

When I did my first three-week-long Detox Diet, I learned to chew my food thoroughly for the first time in my life. I felt more nourished on less food, and I experienced less bloating, gas, and fullness in the several hours after eating. My weight dropped 5 pounds per week and I felt clearer, more energized, and less congested.

Over the past twenty years, I have prescribed this Detox Diet (as a healing diet and catalyst for habit changes) for those with obvious congestion-toxicity concerns, such as people with high blood pressure who are also overweight and stressed, those with arthritis and joint pains, allergies, or recurrent sinus problems, or those with back pains or lymphatic congestion.

Most people experience similar results—a couple of days of transition with occasional fatigue, irritability, hunger, or increased congestion. Usually by the third day they start to feel cleaner, clearer, lighter, stronger, and more present in their body, aware of the way it responds to food and liquid intake. Their symptoms of congestion and pain diminish and even disappear. It is very gratifying for them and me and often represents a long-term change, and it certainly makes my job more enjoyable and rewarding.

OTHER DIETS FOR DETOXIFICATION

The following detoxifying and purifying diet programs cover a wide range of caloric needs to help you tailor a program just right for you. They include the **Detox Diet, Smoothie Cleanse,** and **Juice Cleanse**. These varying programs allow some diversity to help guide you through the most appropriate cleanse depending on your body type and needs, the time of year, the length of time you would like to cleanse, and your individual food sensitivities and caloric needs. The next chapter, Transitional Diets, will help you move out of the Detox Diet or cleansing program

THE NONTOXIC DIET

- Eat organically grown foods whenever possible.

- Drink filtered (or properly purified) water.

- Eat a natural, seasonal cuisine, focusing on fresh foods as much as possible.

- Include fruits, vegetables, whole grains, legumes, nuts, and seeds, and, for omnivarians, some low- or nonfat dairy products (particularly organic yogurt), fresh fish (not shellfish), and organic poultry.

- Rotate foods, especially common allergens such as milk products, eggs, wheat, and yeasted foods. Following a gluten-free diet helps many people.

- Practice food combining, avoiding mixing too many foods per meal.

- Avoid overeating or eating too much food too late in your day.

- Cook in iron, stainless steel, glass, or porcelain cookware.

- Avoid or minimize red meats, cured meats, organ meats, refined foods, canned foods, sugar, salt, saturated fats, coffee, alcohol, and nicotine.

and create a healthy, long-term diet. The specific Lifelong Detox Diet includes a hypoallergenic plan with avoidance of regular use of SNACCs (sugar, nicotine, alcohol, caffeine, and chemicals).

GETTING A PROFESSIONAL EVALUATION

Working with a practitioner's guidance for detoxification can be helpful. This is typically a naturally oriented medical doctor, naturopath, nutritionist, or acupuncturist—obviously a health professional who has had training and experience in detoxification. When I set up an initial personalized detox/cleansing program, I evaluate each individual with a health history, physical exam, biochemical tests, dietary review, and other relevant tests based on the person's needs. These tests could include digestive analyses for function as well as microbes (both normal and abnormal), blood mineral levels, and an evaluation of food-immune, allergy-like reactions through blood. By interpreting the patient's current symptoms and medical problems as a result of diet, lifestyle, and genetic patterns, and by then considering the patient's current health goals, we can create a plan together. As is true with any healing process, the plan must be reevaluated and fine-tuned to the individual to make it work optimally over time.

If the patient is deficient in nutrients and/or energy, she may need a higher-protein, higher-nutrient rebuilding diet—greater nourishment rather than a cleansing program to improve her health. Fatigue, mineral deficiencies, and low organ functions may call for this more supportive, nourishing diet, and not so much detoxifying. However, even in these circumstances, doing a short three-day cleanse or avoiding foods like wheat, sugar, and milk products can help eliminate old debris and prepare the body to build with healthier blocks.

Our individual detox (purifying) programs do change, as our needs often vary with time. For instance, my own personal program has changed in intensity over the decades. Initially, fasts were very powerful, transformative, and healing for me. Now I feel much cleaner most of the time, and I usually notice less effect from a fast. If I do get congested with different foods, travel, or when under stress, a few days of juices or light eating will make a big difference. I ate a low-protein, high-complex-carbohydrate vegetarian diet for a number of years; now my mild detoxification consists of more strengthening protein-vegetable meals. Fresh fish with lots of vegetables satisfies and energizes me more now than it did in the past. My previous higher-starch diet led me to overeat in order to feel nourished. This new diet has let me reduce calories and weight while feeling stronger and healthier. And this too, I am sure, will change over time.

CHOOSING THE RIGHT PROGRAM FOR YOU

Here are a few other tips on which cleanse or detox program to choose, how long to detox, and how to move from one to the other program. The best way to think about them is to see the Detox Diet as the basic plan, moving along to more intensity with the Smoothie Cleanse, and last, the most extreme, the Juice Cleanse. In actuality, water fasting is the most intense, but we do not recommend that here, as it should be done under supervision in most situations and doesn't typically allow one to keep working or working out; it is a rest time.

In our groups, we often use these different levels of the detox programs as stepping stones toward our longer range goal of cleaning up our bodies, losing weight, clearing symptoms, and creating overall healing. Everyone feels lighter and clearer with the feeling of making a fresh start. The transition back into the right diet for each of you is the most important part of the whole process. If you just go back to your old diet (unless it is already very good), it likely isn't worth the whole effort, because your body and health will soon return to that lesser level as well. The key idea for this detoxification process is to come out the other side with more awareness and healthier habits, and then a healthier body. Each of the following programs can also be done exclusively, such as the Detox Diet for two to three weeks, the Smoothie Cleanse for one to two weeks, or the Juice Cleanse for three to ten or more days, all depending on the body state and needs.

A good example of a two- to three-week process can start with the Detox Diet for about a week, then shift over to smoothies and juices, either combined over the day or done exclusively. Many people can combine the liquid cleansing with the Detox Diet, where they do juices through the day, but have a salad or steamed veggies at lunch and/or dinner. As you detox, you will be learning (or really relearning) to listen to your body and adapt as you are instinctually guided. This process is both common and extremely empowering for most participants in my groups. After the cleansing week, you can move back into the Detox Diet for another week. Make sure you are balancing with supplements (see chapter 6), drinking water, and exercising. Next, you can move into the Transition Diets described in chapter 7, and hopefully not back into the bread and cheese, or candy and soda plan. Stay with your transition diet because habits can change just by making good choices and eating good foods. Think about what you can eat, what's right for you, and not what you can't have. Your bowl is not half empty, but half full on the way to flowing over the brim with great health. Good luck and good health!

THE DETOX DIET AND DAILY MENU PLAN

Many thousands of people have successfully benefited from following this simple menu plan. This program can be done for just one day or up to three to four weeks. The diet includes wholesome foods such as whole grains, vegetables, fruits, and teas. It can also be expanded to include dressings, dips, and sauces as well as drinks to help those who would like to follow the diet longer (see recipes in part 3). The Smoothie Cleanse provides added nutritional drinks for those who need more calories and/or protein for energy, weight maintenance, and muscle support. Even adding smoothies to the Detox Diet makes the overall program more caloric and nutritional, and thus prevents weight loss.

However, it also may be less detoxifying. When following a longer-term program, we also suggest adding fish (or other good proteins) to the program if you are active, have hypoglycemia, or just generally need more protein and calories. The added protein helps make this a more balanced diet over time, because the more stringent plan is not completely balanced. Adding some of the blue-green algaes does offer some more nutrients, amino acids, and protein.

THE DETOX DIET DAILY MENU PLAN

Upon rising

2 glasses of water (filtered), 1 glass or both with the juice of half a lemon.

Breakfast

1 piece of fresh fruit (at room temperature), such as an apple, a pear, a banana, a citrus fruit, or some grapes. Chew well, mixing each bite with saliva.

   15 to 30 minutes later: 1 bowl of cooked whole grains—millet, brown rice, amaranth, and quinoa are the best choices. Oatmeal may be used because it is a favorite breakfast grain for many, but it does have some congestive qualities, as do most grains. (We are avoiding the "gluten" grains of wheat, rye, and barley.) For flavoring, use 2 tablespoons of fruit juice, for sweetness, or 1 tablespoon of Better Butter (page 69) with a little sea salt or tamari for a more savory taste.

Lunch (12 to 1 p.m.)

1 to 2 medium bowls of steamed vegetables. Use a variety and include the roots, stems, and greens. For example, potatoes or yams, green beans, broccoli or cauliflower, carrots or beets, asparagus, kale or chard, and cabbage. Add 1 to 2 teaspoons of dressing, such as Better Butter (page 69). Be sure to chew well!

Dinner (5 to 6 p.m.)

Same as lunch. If you feel fatigued or in need of protein, 3 to 4 ounces of fish, poultry, or beans can be added to this meal or, even better, at 3 to 4 p.m.

Beverage breaks for alkaline support (11 a.m. and 3 p.m.)

Drink the water collected from steaming the vegetables. It contains many nutrients and offers a more alkaline balance for the body. A bit of veggie salt or garlic salt can be added to boost flavor. A green powder or buffered vitamin C powder can be mixed in as well (see chapter 6).

Before retiring

Consume no additional foods after dinner. Drink only water and herbal teas.

Note: Eating times are relatively important, especially your last meal; finish eating at 6 p.m. or so, or by nightfall at the latest, if your schedule can't conform. Having that rest from food overnight is important to the detoxification process.

Better Butter

Better Butter spreads easily and is lower in cholesterol and saturated fat than dairy butter. Flaxseed oil can also be used. This recipe is adapted from The New Laurel's Kitchen. MAKES 32 SINGLE-TABLESPOON SERVINGS

1 cup extra virgin olive oil, preferably organic

1 cup (2 sticks) organic butter, at room temperature or melted over low heat

In a glass bowl, combine the olive oil and butter until well mixed. Cover and store in the refrigerator for up to 2 weeks.

SMOOTHIE CLEANSE

The Smoothie Cleanse is a general short-term diet (one to two weeks) of fruit smoothies and vegetable juices and smoothies, which can be supplemented with green products for energy and with protein powder for those who have a higher caloric or protein need.

Adding protein powder to your smoothies is especially important for those who do not want to lose weight, for athletes who don't wish to lower muscle mass, and for those with hypoglycemia (low blood sugar issues). Good-quality protein powders are available from rice, milk (whey proteins), hemp, or soy (organic soy only).

Smoothies are easy to make, are delicious, and only require minimal equipment and preparation. All you need is a blender (unless you wish to squeeze or press your own juices first, which is ideal). You can personalize your smoothie to include your favorite flavors and the protein you need for an active lifestyle, as well as hide potent detoxifiers in these cool, rich drinks.

The basic formula for a smoothie is 1 cup (per person) of liquid such as fruit juice, rice milk, almond milk, organic soy-milk, oat milk, or multi-grain milk. (*Note:* We prefer that you avoid cow's milk for a variety of health-related reasons; however, some people still favor cow's milk and whey protein powder, or goat's milk and its products.) Add a banana plus 1 cup of other fruit, either fresh or frozen, and you have your base drink. Smoothies are so rich and creamy (a half to a whole banana helps with this quality) that you can hide ingredients such as ground flax-seed, wheat germ, flaxseed oil, and protein powders without changing the flavor too much. (This is useful when nourishing your kids with smoothies.) There are other protein powders besides the typical whey or soy; these include rice, hemp, and pea protein. On top of that you can add nutrients such as probiotics (healthy bacteria such as acidophilus), algae, vitamin C, and many other supplements. This is a great benefit to those on the run and for those who have a hard time swallowing supplements.

Drink and chew your smoothies as soon as possible after making them so the ingredients are fresh and have not oxidized. For many more smoothie recipes, see *Smoothies for Life!* and *More Smoothies for Life* by Daniella Chace.

THE SMOOTHIE CLEANSE DAILY MENU PLAN

Upon rising
2 glasses of water (filtered), 1 glass with the juice of half a lemon.

Breakfast
1 piece of fresh fruit (at room temperature), such as an apple, a pear, a banana, an orange, a grapefruit, or grapes. Chew well, mixing each bite with saliva, to awaken your digestion.

15 to 30 minutes later: a smoothie made with fruit and juice or milk alternative. Add ingredients to meet your specific needs, such as protein powder if you are active. Remember to chew your smoothie to mix your saliva with the rich fluid, which helps begin the digestive process.

Lunch (12 to 1 p.m.)
A smoothie or fresh vegetable juice.

Snack (3 p.m.)
A smoothie or fresh vegetable juice.

Dinner (5 to 6 p.m.)
A smoothie or fresh vegetable juice.

Before retiring
Consume no additional foods after dinner. Drink only water and herbal teas.

SAMPLE SMOOTHIE RECIPES

(See part 3 for more smoothie recipes.)

High-Energy Banana Shake

Bananas provide electrolytes and easily absorbed calories to boost energy. SERVES 1

1 cup milk alternative (rice, almond, coconut, hemp, or oat)

1 banana (fresh or frozen)

1 to 2 tablespoons protein powder

Blend all the ingredients in a food processor or blender until smooth. Drink immediately.

Berry Cooler

Berries contain cleansing fiber and antioxidants. Frozen berries create more of a milkshake effect than fresh. Protein powder can be added to this or any smoothie for those who have higher caloric needs. SERVES 1

1 cup milk, milk alternative, or juice

$1/2$ to 1 cup berries (fresh or frozen)

1 to 2 tablespoons protein powder (optional)

1 banana (optional)

Blend all the ingredients in a food processor or blender until smooth. Drink immediately.

Carrot Smoothie

Carrots contain powerful antioxidants and although they cannot be juiced in a blender, carrot juice can be added to any smoothie as a base ingredient. Freshly made carrot juice from your home juicer is best or from the local natural food store (many make fresh juice), or buy freshly bottled juices. If you use bottled vegetable juices, make sure you get them without added sodium.

SERVES 1

1 cup carrot juice (fresh or bottled)

2 tablespoons apple juice

1 tablespoon fresh lemon juice

Ice (optional)

Blend all the ingredients in a food processor or blender until smooth. Drink immediately.

JUICE CLEANSE

This three- to ten-day deeper cleanse is the perfect spring plan for many people. The popular Master Cleanser (page 53) is an integral part of the program, which also may include vegetable juices, fruit juices, and vegetable broths.

The juice cleanse diet is a short-term, effective purifying program consisting of nutrient-rich vegetable and fruit juices. Candidates for this diet are those who want to lose weight, want to increase the rate of toxin clearing, and have lower caloric needs because they are not extremely active.

Regular exercise is still suggested to burn calories and get or stay in shape.

If you haven't experienced fresh juices before, you are in for a big surprise. They are so packed with nutrients and are very energizing. Fruits and vegetables contain easily absorbed vitamins and minerals, calories for immediate energy production, and vital phytonutrients. These naturally occurring plant nutrients protect us from disease, help heal imbalances, and accelerate the healing process.

To make fresh juices, which are superior to bottled juices, you will need a juicer (see page 58). The centrifugal force juicers are easy to clean and extract juice well from the pulp of the plants. If you have an orange juice squeezer, you can make fresh citrus juice. However, investing in a juicer will give you the ability to make your own fresh vegetable juices, which are the most vitally alive.

Juices can be made from one item or are usually a concoction of various fruits or vegetables. For example, apples with lemon and ginger are warming and enhance digestion, while a combination of carrots, celery, and lemon is refreshing and energizing.

It's important to drink freshly made juices as soon as possible (ideally immediately) so the nutrients are not exposed to air and light for very long. Some of the vitamins and phytonutrients can oxidize and be lost over time, ranging from minutes to days.

Additional detoxifying foods can be eaten to vary and simplify the juice cleanse, to extend the cleanse, or if you need to add more fruit and calories. Vegetable soups can be consumed, as can fresh fruits and vegetables such as celery, carrots, jicama, apples, pears, oranges, and so forth. See part 3 for recipes and chapter 4 for more juice ideas. Use in-season and organic fruits and vegetables as much as possible. (See the Seasonal Vegetable Suggestions list on page 66 as well.)

SAMPLE JUICE RECIPES

(See part 3 for more juice recipes.)

Apple Breeze

This refreshing juice is fairly low in calories and rich in nutrients. This is the perfect drink after a steam, yoga, or stretching session. SERVES 1

2 apples, seeded

2 stalks celery

1/4 lemon

Juice all the ingredients according to your machine's instructions. Serve over ice or with a mint leaf or lemon wedge for garnish. Drink immediately.

Lemon Veggie Delight

This light vegetable juice has a sweet edge from the carrots and a bit of zip from the lemon. You can add any greens you happen to have on hand because most greens, such as bok choy (Chinese cabbage), spinach, and garden greens, all taste wonderful with carrot and lemon. SERVES 1

4 carrots

2 stalks celery

4 leaves kale

1 lemon

Juice all the ingredients according to your machine's instructions. Drink immediately.

Fresh Tomato Juice

Use the ripest tomatoes possible. Garden tomatoes are exquisite juiced fresh. SERVES 1

2 medium tomatoes

1/2 red bell pepper

Celery, carrots, yellow or orange bell pepper, onion, 1 to 2 cloves garlic (all optional)

Juice all the ingredients according to your machine's instructions. Drink immediately.

THE JUICE CLEANSE DAILY MENU PLAN

Upon rising
2 glasses of water (filtered), 1 glass with the juice of half a lemon.

Breakfast
3 to 4 (8-ounce) glasses of Master Cleanser (page 53), consumed over the morning, or 1 portion of fresh fruit (at room temperature), such as an apple, a pear, an orange, a grapefruit, or grapes. Chew well, mixing each bite with saliva to awaken your digestion.

Mid-morning
Several (6- to 8-ounce) glasses of fresh fruit or vegetable juice (in place of or after the Master Cleanser). These can be diluted with water, up to half. Apples, grapes, and lemon make a great fruit juice mix. Fresh grapes and freshly made organic grape juice are a good combination.

Lunch (12 to 1 p.m.)
1 (12-ounce) glass of fresh vegetable juice, Master Cleanser, or fruit juice.

Snack (3 p.m.)
6 to 12 ounces of fresh vegetable juice. Carrot, beet, and celery are great together. Some greens, such as kale or spinach, can be added, or an occasional shot of wheatgrass juice. Ginger, garlic, and/or lemon can be added to the vegetable juice.

Dinner (5 to 6 p.m.)
1 (12-ounce) glass of fresh vegetable juice or some vegetable broth, made from fresh vegetables.

Beverage breaks (11 a.m. and 3 p.m.)
Herbal teas or sparkling water.

Before retiring
Consume no additional foods after dinner. Drink only water and/or herbal teas.

Sweet Beet Elixir

Beet roots have been used in many cultures as a detoxifying juice. Beets are rich in potassium, folic acid, glutathione, and phytoesterols. SERVES 1

- 1 to 2 beets, with greens attached, if desired
- 2 stalks celery
- 1 to 2 carrots
- 2 leaves kale
- Carrot, beet greens, and lemon wedge (optional)

Juice all the ingredients according to your machine's instructions. Drink immediately.

Hot Apple Tonic

The pie spice addition to the juice turns it into a comfort drink. Also apple juice is a natural, gentle laxative, soothing to the digestive tract. SERVES 1

- 2 apples, seeded
- ¾ cup boiling water
- Large pinch of apple pie spice

Juice the apples according to your machine's instructions. Pour the juice into a large mug, add the boiling water, and stir in the spice mix. Drink immediately.

Note about detox reactions: Because juice fasting is such a powerful detoxifier, it frequently causes temporary symptoms, including headaches, fatigue, irritability, bad breath, skin odor, skin eruptions, and a white coating on the tongue. These symptoms, which can be unpleasant and uncomfortable, are a sure sign your metabolism is healing. They should pass in a couple of days and are generally replaced with a very pleasant sense of calmness, great energy, and a feeling of satisfaction. Detox symptoms can also occur with other types of elimination diets.

THE LIFELONG DETOX DIET

This is similar to the nontoxic diet. Avoid SNACCs and common reactive foods, such as wheat and cow's milk products, or at most rotate them into your diet every few days. Many people have problems with wheat and dairy products, and sugar. However, to consume a diet void of bread, cheese, or an occasional sweet treat is rather extreme. Just reserve them for special occasions.

That being said, many of these foods are habits and comfort foods, and once we clear them and see that we feel better, have more energy, and stay trimmer, we find it's not that difficult to avoid them and eat healthier foods. The next chapter gives you a more complete picture of moving back into your health-generating diet. There are other diet options in chapter 7.

CHAPTER SIX

Supplements, Activities, and Products for Detoxification

THERE ARE MANY ASPECTS to healthy detoxification. It is important to support all the organs that help us detoxify—the skin, kidneys, colon, liver, and lungs. **Drinking good water** is crucial for flushing toxins. Regular exercise and sweating are also important, as is lymphatic massage. And keeping our bowels moving is necessary to feeling well during detox programs.

Colon cleansing is one of the most important steps in detoxification. The large intestine releases many toxins, and sluggish functioning of this organ can rapidly produce general body toxicity. During any detox program, most people will incorporate some colon cleansing. Helpful products include laxatives, fiber, and colon detox supplements such as chia seeds or psyllium seed husks alone or mixed with other agents such as aloe vera powder, bentonite clay, and acidophilus culture. Enemas using water, herbs, or even diluted coffee (although popular in some detox programs, I do not recommend this latter process, which is said to stimulate liver cleansing) may be used. A series of colonic water irrigations (best performed by a trained professional with filtered water and sterile equipment and now referred to as colon hydrotherapy) can be the focal point of a detox program accompanied by a cleansing diet and fiber supplements.[1] There is controversy over the use

SIMPLE SUPPLEMENTS FOR THE DETOX DIET

Multiple vitamin-mineral (one-a-day type)
1 tablet or capsule after breakfast

Antioxidant combination
1 to 2 caps or tabs twice daily, between meals

**Vitamin C or buffered powdered vitamin C with minerals
(calcium, magnesium, and potassium)**
1 tab or cap of 500 to 1,000 mg vitamin C, or $1/2$ to 1 teaspoon twice daily of powder mixed into liquid

Calcium-magnesium capsule or tablet
1 to 3 caps at bedtime or 1 to 2 for muscle cramps to be utilized if the buffered vitamin C powder is not being used

Blue-green algae, spirulina, or chlorella
2 to 4 tabs or caps after breakfast and lunch (double the number of tabs for chlorella because they are smaller)

Herbal colon tablets or laxative tea
1 to 2 tabs twice daily in the morning and evening, or about $1/2$ to 1 cup of tea, morning and evening (varies depending on individual sensitivity)

Herbal extracts can also be used to support or balance other body systems or to enhance energy. Siberian or other ginsengs, echinacea for immune support, and ginger for circulation are options. Review the lists of herbs later in this chapter.

of colon irrigation, so if you choose that route, please make sure you go to an experienced practitioner. Whatever the method, keeping the bowels moving is key to feeling well during detoxification.

Regular exercise is also very important during detoxification (as always) because it stimulates sweating and encourages elimination through the skin. Exercise also improves our general metabolism and helps overall with detoxification. For this reason, regular aerobic exercise is key to maintaining a nontoxic body, especially when we indulge in various substances such as sugar or alcohol. Because exercise releases toxins in the body, it is important to incorporate adequate fluids, antioxidants, vitamins, and minerals.

Regular bathing cleanses the skin of toxins that have been released and opens the pores for further elimination, and this is particularly beneficial during detoxification. Saunas and sweats are commonly used to enhance skin elimination.[2] Dry brushing the skin with an appropriate skin brush before bathing is also suggested to invigorate the skin and cleanse away old cells. Massage therapy (especially lymphatic or deep tissue) stimulates elimination and body functions and promotes relaxation. Clearing generalized tensions also makes for a more complete detoxification.

Resting, relaxation, and recharging are also important to this rejuvenation process. During the detox process, we may need more rest, quiet time, and sleep, although most commonly we have more energy and function better on less sleep than before. Relaxation exercises help our bodies rebalance themselves, as our minds and our attitudes stop interfering with our natural homeostasis. The practice of yoga combines quiet yet powerful exercises with breath awareness and regulation, allowing increased flexibility and relaxation.

Certain **supplements** are appropriate for some detoxification programs. However, general supplementation may be less important in this detox program than with the specific detox plans for alcohol, caffeine, and nicotine, when more nutrients can ease withdrawal symptoms. (These specific substance detoxification programs are discussed in part 2.)

For straight juice cleansing or water fasts, we usually do not recommend many supplements; however, some nutrients or herbs to stimulate the detoxification process may be helpful. Examples include potassium, extra fiber with olive oil to clear toxins from the colon, sodium alginate from seaweeds to bind heavy metals, and apple cider vinegar in water (1 tablespoon vinegar in 8 ounces hot water) to help reduce mucus. Blue-green algae, chlorella, and spirulina are nutrient-rich foods that may supply physical and mental energy. For people who begin with transition diets, a specialized nutrient program may help neutralize toxins and support elimination. With weight loss (for detoxers who are overweight), toxins stored in the fat will need to be mobilized and cleared—thus, more water, fiber, and antioxidant nutrients can help handle this.

The supplement program used for general detoxification (with additional support to reduce nutrient deficiency during detox) is outlined in the table at the end of this chapter. It includes a low-dosage multiple vitamin-mineral supplement to fulfill the basic nutritional requirements during the transitional diet. The B vitamins, particularly niacin, are also important, as are minerals such as zinc, calcium, magnesium, and potassium. The antioxidant nutrients include vitamins C and E, beta-carotene or mixed carotenoids, vitamin A, zinc, and selenium. Some authorities believe higher amounts of vitamin A (10,000 IU), mixed carotenoids (25,000 to 50,000 IU), vitamin C (8 to 12 g), selenium (300 to 400 mcg), and vitamin E (1,000 to 1,200 IU) are helpful during detoxification to neutralize the free radicals. This may be more than most people really need.

The liver is our most important detoxification organ. The B vitamins, especially B$_3$ (niacin) and B$_6$ (pyridoxine), vitamins A and C, zinc, calcium, vitamin E and selenium, and L-cysteine are also needed to support liver detoxification. Milk thistle herb (often sold as silymarin or *Silybum marianum*) has also been shown to aid liver detoxification and repair.[3]

Several **amino acids** improve or support detoxification, particularly cysteine and methionine, which contain sulfur. L-cysteine supplies sulfhydryl groups, which help prevent oxidation and bind heavy metals such as mercury; vitamin C and selenium aid this process

---

SAMPLE DETOX FORMULA

Echinacea
Cayenne pepper
Parsley leaf
Goldenseal root
Garlic
Licorice root
Yellow dock root

Obtain powders (or ground herbs) in equal amounts for all of the above except cayenne, for which you should get half. Mix and put into size "00" capsules. Take two capsules two or three times daily between meals. Drink lots of water with this as well.

---

as well. Cysteine is the precursor to glutathione—our most important cellular detoxifier—which counters many chemicals and carcinogens. Glutathione is used by the detoxification enzyme *glutathione peroxidase*, which works to prevent peroxidation of lipids and decrease toxins such as smoke, radiation, auto exhaust, chemicals, drugs, and other carcinogens. *Glutathione reductase* is the enzyme that regenerates glutathione to its active, reduced form.

Glycine is a secondary helper because it is one of the three amino acids that comprise glutathione. Glycine decreases the toxicity of substances such as phenols or benzoic acid (a food preservative). This can be taken as the supplement TMG (trimethylglycine). Glutamine is also

CLEANSING HERBS

- **Garlic**—blood cleanser, may lower blood fats and cholesterol, natural antibiotic and antimicrobial for bacteria, yeasts, parasites, viral infections

- **Red clover blossoms**—blood cleanser, good during convalescence and healing

- **Echinacea**—lymph cleanser, improves lymphocyte and phagocyte actions, immunity supporter, antimicrobial

- **Dandelion root**—liver and blood cleanser, diuretic, filters toxins, a tonic

- **Chaparral**—strong blood cleanser, with possibilities for use in cancer therapy

- **Cayenne pepper**—blood and tissue purifier, increases fluid elimination and perspiration, a natural stimulant

- **Cascara sagrada**—a colon cleanser and bowel tonic

- **Gingerroot**—stimulates circulation and perspiration, relieves congestion, helps nausea

- **Licorice root**—the "great detoxifier," biochemical balancer, mild laxative, supports immune function, stomach soother (for inflammation/irritation)

- **Yellow dock root**—skin, blood, and liver cleanser, contains vitamin C and iron

- **Burdock root**—skin and blood cleanser, diuretic, increases perspiration, improves liver function, antibacterial and antifungal properties

- **Sarsaparilla root**—blood and lymph cleanser, contains saponins (which reduce microbes and toxins)

- **Prickly ash bark**—good for nerves and joints, anti-infectious

- **Oregon grape root**—skin and colon cleanser, blood purifier, liver stimulant

- **Parsley leaf**—diuretic, flushes kidneys, breath freshener

- **Goldenseal root**—blood, liver, kidney, and skin cleanser, stimulates detoxification, antimicrobial

important in helping heal the GI tract as well as reduce cravings for sugar and alcohol, should they occur. Other amino acids that may have mild detoxifying effects are methionine, tyrosine, and taurine.

As mentioned earlier, **fiber also supports detoxification and elimination.** Psyllium seed husks (often combined with other detox nutrients, such as pectin, aloe vera, alginates, and/or colon herbs) help cleanse mucus along the small intestine, create bulk in the colon, and pull toxins from the gastrointestinal tract. When fiber is combined with 1 or 2 tablespoons of olive oil, it helps bind toxins and reduce the absorption of fats and some basic minerals. Psyllium husks also reduce absorption of the olive oil itself, which is important in reducing calories and binding any fat-soluble chemicals that may have been released. An option then involves taking 1 to 2 teaspoons each of psyllium husks and bran several times daily (with meals and at bedtime) along with 1 teaspoon of olive oil to help detoxify the colon. Some people find psyllium husks to be irritating. People generally start with 1 teaspoon a day and build up from there to prevent gas and gut discomfort. Another option, and possibly even a better choice, is chia seed. Chia has a higher nutrient level, especially of omega-3 oils, which provide further benefit. It also holds more water and has a healing component for irritated colon mucosa. Acidophilus and other beneficial bacteria (probiotics) in the colon neutralize some toxins, reduce the metabolism of other microbes, and lessen colon toxicity. Supplemental probiotics can be added to the detox program. There are many products in the marketplace, most now containing billions of organisms per capsule. Most require refrigeration for protection.

WATER

Remember, water is crucial to any type of detox program for diluting and eliminating toxin accumulations. It is probably our most important detoxifier because it helps us clean through our skin and kidneys, and improves our sweating with exercise. One of my favorite sayings is, "Dilution is the solution to pollution." Eight to ten glasses a day (depending on body size and activity level, as well as local climate) of clean, filtered water are suggested. Some authorities suggest using distilled water during detox programs, as its lack of minerals draws other particles (nutrients and toxins) to it. However, since distilled water may alter our biochemical and electrical balance, drinking purified or clean spring water is preferred. Two or three glasses of water 30 to 60 minutes before each meal (and at night) will help flush toxins during our body's natural elimination time.

Water Tips
- Lack of water as dehydration is a primary cause of daytime fatigue and headaches.

- Seventy-five percent of Americans are chronically dehydrated, particularly the elderly.

- The thirst mechanism is often so weak, it can be mistaken for hunger.

- Even mild dehydration will slow down one's metabolism by as much as 3 percent, and more severe dehydration by 5 percent.

- Drinking water improved weight loss in overweight women; those who drank more water lost more weight than the women who had low to no water intake.[4]

- Preliminary research indicates eight to ten glasses of water a day could significantly ease back and joint pain for many sufferers.

- A mere 2 percent drop in body water can diminish cognitive function and mood, plus trigger fuzzy short-term memory, trouble with basic math, and difficulty focusing on the computer screen or on a printed page.[5]

How Much Water Should You Drink?

There is some controversy over how much we really need daily, but we think for most people it's healthy to drink at least 2 quarts, which is 64 ounces (eight 8-ounce glasses). Yet, read on to see all the important factors in determining how much water you really need.

Drying Effects

Many factors affect your body's need for water. You may need more or less drinking water depending on lifestyle, diet, medications, and so forth. For example, if you eat a lot of drying foods such as breads, crackers, salty foods, and high-fat or sugary foods, you will need more water just to process these foods through your digestive system. Also, if you take in caffeine and other diuretics such as coffee, espresso, tea (black and green), chocolate, or caffeinated sodas (such as Coke, Pepsi, or Mountain Dew), you are flushing water and electrolytes out of your system and must replace the fluid and nutrients. Many lifestyle choices can be drying, such as drinking alcohol (wine, beer, and hard alcohol), smoking, recreational drugs and over-the-counter drugs, chewing tobacco, and cigars. Also, if your environment is dry because you use high heat in your house or car or heavy blankets or sweat at night, then you will have an increased need for water.

Hydrating Habits

On the other hand, if you eat a lot of fresh fruits and vegetables and drink high-water-content juices and other liquids, such as almond and other nut milks, or soy and rice milks, your daily need for water will be lower. Eating cooked whole grains and legumes adds some further hydration; legumes are beans, peas, and lentils. They are full of beneficial soluble fiber such as gels and pectins that help hold on to water in your intestines, allowing your body to

GENERAL CLASSIFICATION OF HERBS USEFUL IN DETOXIFICATION*

Blood Cleansers
Echinacea
Red clover
Dandelion
Burdock
Yellow dock
Oregon grape root

Laxatives/Colon Cleansers
Cascara sagrada
Buckthorn
Dandelion
Yellow dock
Rhubarb root
Senna leaf
Licorice

Diuretics
Parsley
Yarrow
Cleavers
Horsetail
Corn silk
Uva ursi
Juniper berries

Skin Cleansers (Diaphoretics)**
Burdock
Oregon grape
Yellow dock
Goldenseal
Boneset
Elder flowers
Peppermint
Cayenne pepper
Gingerroot

Antibiotics
Garlic
Myrrh
Prickly ash
Wormwood
Echinacea
Propolis
Clove
Eucalyptus

Anticatarrhals***
Echinacea
Boneset
Goldenseal
Sage
Hyssop
Garlic
Yarrow

* Not usually used with fasting or juice cleansing, but as supplements to dietary detoxification—using herbs alone may be the most productive in some detoxification programs. A program that includes juice cleansing and specific herbal therapies is best designed by an experienced practitioner in natural medicine and detoxification.

** Diaphoretics increase perspiration.

*** Anticatarrhals help eliminate mucus.

reabsorb water before it passes through you. Also, essential fatty acids (EFAs) from fish and plants, such as flax and borage, are important dietary nutrients for water absorption into the cells.

Athletes' Water Needs

Most people sweat when they work out and lose a considerable amount of water and electrolytes through their pores. A general guideline for water replacement is 1 quart of electrolyte water (32 ounces) for every hour of heavy exercise. That includes hiking, running, swimming, lifting weights, tennis, yard work, cleaning house, and so forth. And during summer or if you live in a generally hotter climate, you will need additional fluids.

WHAT ARE ELECTROLYTES?

The salts or ionized forms of potassium, magnesium, sodium, calcium, and chloride are electrical conductors necessary for nerve and heart function, as well as for supporting hydration. I suggest trace mineral liquids added to water for many of my patients. We need these minerals, especially the electrolytes, to help the water move into the cells and tissues, where real hydration and health are crucial. The aging process is partly dependent on intracellular (inside the cells) water, with young, healthy people showing about 60 percent intracellular water and

unhealthy elders closer to 40 percent. From consistent measurements of body composition at my office, we believe this hydration marker is key to monitoring long-term health and vitality.

Electrolyte Replacement Drinks

Don't fall for those inferior sugary, chemical-food colored mixes such as Gatorade. There are several high-quality electrolyte drinks and powder mixes now available. Knudsen makes an electrolyte replacement drink called Recharge, which is a mix of fruit juice, water, and electrolytes. It is available in orange, lemon, and fruit punch flavors. Also, powders like Power Paks from Trace Mineral Research or the popular Emergen-C products from Alacer Corporation and their inexpensive electrolyte powder called Electro-Mix are good choices as well. These products contain no food coloring, sugar, or calories.

Natural Electrolyte Replacement

Fruits and vegetables are rich in natural electrolytes. Drink smoothies, fresh fruit juices, or bottled or canned concentrates of organic fruit juices. Also, nuts and seeds contain loads of nutrients, and they do have good oils (and calories), so eating a handful or so provides good fuel for activity or recharging after exercise.

GENERAL DETOXIFICATION NUTRIENT PROGRAM—DAILY AMOUNTS

Most of the following nutrients are found in a basic multiple vitamin-mineral formula.

Nutrient	Amount	Nutrient	Amount
Water	2.5 to 3 qt	Selenium	300 mcg
Fiber	20 to 40 g	Silicon	100 mg
Vitamin A	4,000 to 6,000 IU	Vanadium	300 mcg
Beta-carotene or mixed carotenoids	15,000 to 30,000 IU	Zinc	30 mg
Vitamin D	400 to 2,000 IU	**Optional**	
Vitamin E	400 to 1,000 IU	L-amino acids (general blend)	500 to 1,000 mg
Vitamin K	200 mcg	Extra virgin olive oil	3 to 6 teaspoons
Thiamine (B$_1$)	10 to 25 mg	L-cysteine	500 to 1,000 mg
Riboflavin (B$_2$)	10 to 25 mg	Liquid chlorophyll	2 to 4 teaspoons
Niacinamide (B$_3$)	50 mg	DL-methionine	250 to 500 mg
Niacin (B$_3$)	50 to 2,000 mg*	Apple cider vinegar	1 to 2 tablespoons
Pantothenic acid (B$_5$)	250 to 500 mg	L-glycine	250 to 500 mg
Pyridoxine (B$_6$)	10 to 25 mg	L-glutamine	500 to 1,000 mg
Cobalamin (B$_{12}$)	50 to 100 mcg	Psyllium or chia seeds	2 to 4 teaspoons or 8 to 10 caps
Folic acid	400 to 800 mcg	Flaxseed oil	1 to 2 teaspoons or 2 to 4 caps
Biotin	200 mcg	Acidophilus/ Probiotic culture	more than 2 billion organisms per day
Vitamin C	1 to 4 g	Detox formula herbs:	4 to 6 capsules echinacea, yellow dock, goldenseal, garlic, parsley, licorice, cayenne pepper
Bioflavonoids	250 to 500 mg		
Calcium	600 to 850 mg		
Chromium	200 mcg		
Copper	2 mg		
Iodine	150 mcg		
Magnesium	300 to 500 mg		
Manganese	5 to 10 mg		
Molybdenum	300 mcg		
Potassium	300 to 500 mg		

GENERAL DETOXIFICATION NUTRIENT PROGRAM

The program on page 84 has ranges of most nutrients and supplies the body with the vitamins and minerals, and amino and fatty acids, that support our tissues, a healthy liver, and the overall process of detoxification. See chapter 5 for specific programs for the Detox Diet.

Endnotes

1. Michael F. Picco, "Consumer Health: Colon Cleansing," Mayo Clinic, 2011. www .mayoclinic.com/health/colon-cleansing/ AN00065 (accessed November 10, 2011).

2. David E. Root, "Sauna Detoxification: A Treatment Program for Veterans Who Have Symptoms Associated with Chemical Exposure." Presentation Abstract at the Third International Conference on Chemical Contamination and Human Detoxification, September 22–23, 2005, Hunter College, New York, NY.

3. Laurie Barclay, "De-liver Me from Evil. Liver Detoxification—Fact or Fad?" WebMD, 2011. http://men.webmd.com/features/liver-detoxification—fact-fad (accessed November 10, 2011); C. Loguercio and D. Festi, "Silybin and the Liver: From Basic Research to Clinical Practice." *World Journal of Gastroenterology* 17, no. 18 (May 14, 2011): 2288–301.

4. J.D. Stookey, F. Constant, B.M. Popkin, and C.D. Gardner, "Drinking Water Is Associated with Weight Loss in Overweight Dieting Women Independent of Diet and Activity," *Obesity* 16, no. 11 (November 2008): 2481–8. www .ncbi.nlm.nih.gov/pubmed/18787524.

5. B.M. Popkin, K.E. D'Anci, and I.H. Rosenberg, "Water, Hydration and Health," National Institute of Health, www.ncbi.nlm.nih.gov/pmc/ articles/PMC2908954 (accessed November 10, 2011).

CHAPTER SEVEN
Transitional Diets

TRANSITIONING TO YOUR NEW DAILY DIET

As you transition back to your daily diet you may want to make more changes to create a satisfying diet along with some comfort foods and occasional treats without reintroducing too many toxins. This can be a simple and fun process with a little guidance and a few tips. Transitioning from each of the specific detox cleanses or diet plans has its own considerations. The following tips should help you add foods back into your diet through the transition phase.

The Detox Diet
With this diet you have already been eating some whole grains and vegetables and now your diet can expand to include a wider variety of whole grains such as millet, quinoa, and brown rice. Also, you can now increase protein and good oil foods such as fish, nuts and seeds, avocado, beans, and healthy oils such as flaxseed oil and extra virgin olive oil. See the menu plan on page 98.

The Smoothie Cleanse
Start by adding protein powder to your smoothies if you haven't already. Rice protein is a good choice, with other options being soy (organic and non-GMO whenever possible), or even whey (milk extract) powder, which tends to

be better tolerated than whole cow's milk. Nut butters can also be added to smoothies to increase the protein and oil content. Then add more fruits and raw or steamed vegetables into your meal plan. Over several days of the Smoothie Cleanse, you can begin adding whole grains, beans, fish, some nuts and seeds, and healthy oils back into your diet.

The Juice Cleanse Program

Transition slowly by adding pureed fruit (or chew very thoroughly) such as applesauce, berry puree, and fruit smoothies into your plan. During this phase you can also start eating a variety of steamed vegetables, especially steamed greens, plus some light salads with olive oil and lemon or balsamic vinegar. Again, remember to chew well. Start by adding small amounts of protein (protein powder) to the smoothies; this gets your digestive tract prepared for heavier foods. Do this for at least two days, and then you can begin to eat cooked whole grains, fish, beans, seeds, and oils again. Sprouted beans and seeds are also good sources of protein.

Many people who follow a detox diet will find that allergic symptoms disappear during their program. This may be because a food that caused some reaction was removed from the diet. **The most common allergens are what I call "The Sensitive Seven": wheat, cow's milk, sugar, corn, soy, eggs, and peanuts** (of course, this includes any products made from these foods). Wait to reintroduce these items into your diet until you have

first added back in vegetables, fruits, fish, legumes (except soy and peanuts), whole grains, and some nuts and seeds, such as almonds, filberts, and sunflower seeds. At a later time, you can add the Sensitive Seven foods into the diet one at a time, and watch for any reaction. This way you'll be able to identify any food sensitivities. This is true even for other common foods like almonds or potatoes, and even garlic and kidney beans. Awareness of your body and any reactions to a food or meal is a valuable process for what you have already invested your time and energy.

Evaluating Food Reactions

Here's how you do food challenges to test for reactivity. Choose one of the common sensitive foods. Eat small amounts at first and see if there's any reaction. Then, work up to eating more of that particular food over the coming days. If you still feel fine, you are probably not reacting to that food. Then you can try adding the next food back into your diet and so on. Because of many factors, reactions may not be clear and you still may have questions. Typically, when you have avoided a reactive food, you will show a more significant and clearer reaction when you bring it back into your diet. However, sometimes if you are mildly reactive, it may take a few exposures to notice any reactions from the cumulative effect. You may feel more tired or exprience digestive upset (common with wheat reintroduction), nasal congestion, or a return of other allergy symptoms.

With the most congesting foods, like meats and dairy products, try only small amounts at first (including goat's milk and cheeses). If you feel tired or have digestive upset, sinus stuffiness, or other areas of mucus production, then you may be reacting to that food. If these reactions occur, you should avoid the reactive foods for at least a couple of weeks before rechallenging yourself again. If it's difficult to figure out what you are reacting to, you may want to get a food allergy (antibody) blood test to help you identify which foods are triggering your reactions. These tests vary in their accuracy (or more often, their clinical relevance), yet they can be quite helpful for some people. You can read more about this process and these tests in my book, *The False Fat Diet*.

ADDING PROTEIN BACK INTO YOUR DIET

Slowly reintroduce protein into your diet. It can take several days for your body to get used to more protein and other heavier foods coming in, especially after a juice or smoothie cleanse. Your digestive tract will respond to the protein foods such as beans, peas, and lentils, and even more so with meats and dairy foods by secreting additional hydrochloric acid and digestive enzymes specific to proteins. For example, if you ate a big bowl of chili or a large serving of meat right after a cleansing diet, you may not be able to digest it well, which generally results in gas and constipation, and a very heavy feeling in your body. Some people have a harder time digesting animal foods with a higher fat content, which include red meats, poultry, fish, cheese, or eggs. In this case, supplementing with hydrochloric acids (HCl as betaine hydrochloride, often combined with pepsin, a protein digestant) and/or digestive enzymes may be necessary. Digestive enzymes help break down the carbohydrates, fats, and protein in your diet while HCl helps break down fat and protein. Enzyme supplements and HCl are available from natural food markets, or these supplements may be prescribed by nutritionists and nutritional doctors.

EATING GRAINS AGAIN

Whole grains such as amaranth, oats, millet, quinoa, and brown rice are complex carbohydrates rich in nutrients and fiber. Start with just one serving a day and slowly add whole grains back into your diet, up to three or four servings. If you tend to be a carbohydrate overeater and are watching your weight, you may wish to limit your grains and go even more slowly in bringing them back into your regular diet. I do better this way in controlling my weight. Overall, grains are healthy, high-fiber foods with decent nutritional value, and this supports good elimination. On the other hand, as stated, you may want to limit your dietary grains; some people do best without any in their diet.

If you need to maintain or gain weight, you may want to eat more grains, as well as nuts and seeds. In general, we suggest most people limit their bread and baked good (all made from grains) intake, because there are many healthier choices in the food chain. We suggest you avoid wheat products as long as you can. Yet, good whole-grain dishes are an important part of a healthier, balanced, and more vegetarian, earth-based diet. See part 3 for a few simple and delicious whole-grain recipes.

REINTRODUCING BEANS, PEAS, LENTILS, NUTS, AND SEEDS

Legumes are nutritious partly because they contain so much soluble and insoluble fiber (plus protein and complex carbohydrate), which helps release calories into your bloodstream slowly, allowing time to burn those calories as energy and thus avoid fat storage. But all that fiber is hard for some people to digest, so you may want to take digestive enzymes for the first week or two you are eating those foods again. There's even a product called Beano that helps digest the oligosaccharides in beans. Also, many beans, lentils, nuts, and seeds can be sprouted in your own kitchen. **Sprouting them makes them much easier to digest and more nourishing.** Sprouting activates the plant seed and creates a live growing food, increases protein levels, and makes them easier to digest. There are also sprouted grain and bean products available in natural food stores.

HOW TO CONTINUE AVOIDING SNACCS

Now that you have weaned yourself off of the SNACCs (sugar, nicotine, alcohol, caffeine, and chemicals), you'll want to protect yourself from overdoing them as you transition back into your daily diet. However, certain challenges may arise as you face old routines that once included these substances. Watch these cues so that you lessen your risk of becoming rehabituated to any SNACCs.

Ideally, you will find alternatives to replace them if that is needed. But if you choose to have a cup of coffee or an occasional drink, you can rotate them into your diet and partake in each as a special treat rather than a daily addictive habit, and then you can still maintain your good health. Your body will be able to detoxify these chemicals given the breaks from them. Remember, it's the daily and long-term use and abuse of these substances/drugs that lead to most of their deleterious effects, much as unhealthy aspects of our diets, such as high fat, high calories, and low fiber take decades to cause increases in cancer and cardiovascular problems.

Let's just look at sugar as an example. Now that you have been avoiding it, your taste buds may be more sensitive to sweet foods. You may find candies and sugar-laden foods taste awfully sweet and you may no longer desire them at all; you likewise may appreciate more the natural sweetness of an apple, some cherries, or a carrot. If you do choose to indulge in

Quality Animal Foods

Poultry—Choose organic, free-range, no hormones, no antibiotics birds. Wild game birds are exceptionally healthy as they have a higher level of essential fatty acids due to their natural diet of fruits, seeds, berries, and insects.

Beef—Look for organic, grass-fed, no hormones, no antibiotics beef. When cattle are fattened on corn, the composition of their meat changes drastically. The saturated fat and cholesterol levels go up and the healthy essential fatty acid levels come down.

Dairy—Dairy products should be free of bovine growth hormone ("no rBGH"), antibiotics, and genetically modified organisms ("non-GMO"). Also look for "organic" on milk, cheese, sour cream, yogurt, kefir, and butter. Many of the most toxic chemicals are stored in fat, and since most dairy products have fats (other than nonfat), these chemicals are passed on to us.

Eggs—Buy free-range and organic eggs. You can go a step further and look for "omega-3 fatty acids" on the carton, which tells you the chickens were fed flaxseed. Poultry convert flaxseed into essential fatty acids that end up in the eggs, making them even more nutritious.

Fish—Choose smaller, younger wild fish (salmon, sardines, anchovies, mackerel, herring, shad, snapper), when possible, as they've had less time to accumulate toxins and are rich in essential fatty acids, while farmed varieties are typically low in those beneficial oils and are often fed genetically engineered soybean feed, which is higher in herbicides and other chemical residues. Canned tuna is usually yellow fin, which is fairly large, but albacore tuna is smaller, and the healthier choice. Skipjack, or light tuna, appears to have even lower mercury levels than other tunas. Also be aware that farmed fish may be injected with Red Dye #40 if their flesh appears too pale to be marketable.

something a little sweet you can choose from healthier options. See example recipes in part 3.

Coffee is another issue. Many people love their daily cup-of-joe ritual. Yet, it's wisest to have a healthy and nonhabitual relationship with any of the SNACCs. If you like coffee and the effects of caffeine, try to use that as wisely as possible and take regular coffee breaks, as in the occasional break from coffee and caffeine.

For those who do decide to enjoy an occasional cigarette, make sure your tobacco is high quality, organic, and free of chemicals. The manufacturers of most tobacco products use hundreds of chemicals in the processing of the tobacco, many of which are harmful and toxic. Also, the papers that wrap the tobacco into a cigarette are treated with chemicals that are known toxins. One company that offers nontoxic tobacco is American Spirit Organic Tobacco and another, called Rizla, makes chemical-free paper from rice.

To completely avoid chemicals, you'll want to stay away from processed meats such as salami, bologna, hot dogs, and bacon. Be sure to read labels for MSG, nitrates, preservatives, sugar, and food coloring, most of which you want to avoid. Choose healthier alternatives such as veggie dogs, a beef-like product made from soy. In fact, just about every meat product is now available in a soy form, including salami and Canadian bacon. Also, there are organic, nitrate-free turkey and chicken hot dogs and ground meats for

burgers and meat loaf; thus, healthier options and choices are widely available.

There are also many options and substitutes for cow's milk products, including rice, almond, coconut, and soy bases used to make milks, cheeses, and ice creams. If you do want cow's milk and other animal products, choose higher quality animal products such as organic milk and cheeses.

FROM SIMPLE TO COMPLEX CARBOHYDRATES

Refined flour breaks down in our digestive tracts into sugar within minutes and more quickly than whole-grain products. So if you really want to avoid sugar, you'll want to limit the simple carbohydrates found in refined flour products, including white bread, pasta, bagels, pretzels, many cereals, crackers, doughnuts, cakes, pies, and so forth. If you read the labels, most of these products also have added sugars. It's easy to find healthier whole-wheat and whole-grain alternatives of most baked goods these days, yet it can be a little more difficult to find baked goods with low sugars. You'll need to read food labels to find the healthiest products.

Avoid hydrogenated oil products, including margarines, many packaged baked goods, most crackers and cookies, and fried foods, especially commercial potato and corn chips, which contain partially hydrogenated vegetable oils. As with baked goods, there are healthier versions of chips using organic ingredients and olive oil; there are even baked chips that are not fried.

SUGAR ALTERNATIVES

Sugar is one of the most commonly addictive substances and one of the most damaging because of the level in which it is used. The other extreme is synthetic sweeteners such as aspartame and saccharin. Synthetic sweeteners are made in laboratories by chemical companies and have been linked to brain tumors and bladder cancer. The CDC (Centers for Disease Control) gets more complaints about these chemical sweeteners than any other food products from people who have had headaches and joint pain after ingesting them. We recommend you avoid these toxins.

However, there are delicious alternatives to sugar, such as barley malt syrup, brown rice syrup, xylitol, and stevia, a natural, low-calorie sweet herbal leaf available in powders and liquids. Also you can replace sugar in baking with pureed dates or prunes, which make chewy moist cookies, or applesauce, which replaces the sugar and the fat in a recipe. There are many wonderful baking books to help guide you.

WHAT TO EAT TO STAY HEALTHY

Eat foods in their whole form, as unprocessed as possible, just as nature made them. Every step away from the whole food is a drop in vitality and nourishment. Choose brown rice instead of white rice, steel-cut oats rather than minute oatmeal, whole fruit rather than fruit juice, and so forth. Buy or grow the purest food possible.

Shop your farmers' market if there's one in your area. Use organic produce, grains, and animal products, especially butter, whenever you can. Try to eat at least five to seven servings of fresh vegetables and fruits every day. The focus of a healthy diet is fresh vegetables, balanced with other whole foods. Search out the highest quality fish in your area. Avoid the large fish (examples: swordfish, tuna, and shark), which may contain more ocean toxins, such as mercury; also, avoid farmed fish, which test higher for mercury and other chemicals. Instead, eat albacore tuna, wild salmon, and small fish, such as sardines.

Daily Oil
Extra virgin olive oil is our favorite oil for cooking and salad dressings. It is a clean choice. Extra virgin means the oil came from the very first press of the olives, and typically no chemicals are used in that process, otherwise, buy organic oils. Choose oils that are fresh and store them in a cool, dark place. When oils are exposed to light, oxygen, or heat they can quickly become rancid. You'll know they have gone bad

when they smell fishy or like Play-Doh. Once they have been oxidized, they are rancid and unhealthy for consumption. If that occurs, toss them out and buy some fresh oils for your home.

Plant Foods and Their Phytonutrients

Plant foods are beans, peas, lentils, vegetables, fruits, grains, nuts, seeds, and squashes. They are naturally rich in nutrients and fiber and contain no cholesterol. Most people have a few favorite plant foods they eat on a regular basis, so finding your favorites will help you make them a part of your daily diet. Keeping a bowl of fresh fruit or sliced-up vegetables encourages us to grab a healthy snack when we're busy. Also, making dishes ahead of time is quite helpful to healthy nourishment;

for example, preparing a lentil soup or vegetable chili on the weekend to have on hand during a busy workweek is a habit that will save you money and time during the week. Having the right foods available for our meals or for whenever we're hungry is the best way to stick to a healthy diet. Making your own protein bars with whole oats, barley malt syrup, and soy or rice flour could save you a lot of money, and you can make them with your favorite nuts, sunflower seeds, dried fruits, or even a handful of organic, naturally sweetened chocolate chips. You can also replace the fat and sugar with healthier alternatives so that your personally designed protein bars can have all the ingredients you need to keep your energy up, keep you burning fat, and even satisfy your sweet tooth. See part 3 for phytonutrient-dense recipes.

Nutrient-Dense Foods

Some foods have so many vitamins and minerals that they are almost a dietary supplement; such foods include seaweeds and nutritional yeast. **Seaweeds** include nori, hijiki, arame, kombu, and dulse and have many minerals from the ocean water. Buy seaweed salads that just need water to reconstitute, use the nori to make sushi, and try adding a piece of kombu to your soups to add flavor and nutrients. One easy way to get seaweed nutrients is to buy a bottle of dried seaweed seasoning and add a sprinkle to your grain dishes or to top off your salad. **Nutritional yeast** contains high amounts of B vitamins and some trace minerals as well. It's a cheesy-tasting dried product that comes in flakes or powder, and tastes great on popcorn, on corn tortillas with a little butter, and in macaroni and cheese.

PHYSICAL SUPPORT DURING YOUR TRANSITION

As you start incorporating more physical activity into your daily routine, you will increase your caloric needs. So do this slowly and gently over a two-week period to give your body time to adjust. Yoga and stretching will help awaken your body after your cleanse (and during as well) and assist in the last stage of cleansing. Deep stretching will massage the internal organs, helping to move out old fluids and bring in fresh blood containing nutrients and oxygen. Also, continuing with steams, Epsom salt baths, and dry brushing of the skin will help your body release those deeper layers of toxins through the completion phase of your detoxification program. Of course, massage is great during detoxifying diets.

THE TRANSITIONAL DIETS

The Hypoallergenic, Long-Term Detox Diet

Those who have been diagnosed with food allergies or sensitivities or those suspecting they may be suffering from any food reactions can now test their hypothesis. After cleansing you can assess how you respond to individual foods by reintroducing them one at a time. Even if you have not considered that you may have food reactions, you may have had mystery symptoms that disappeared during your cleanse. In this case, you should take advantage of this transition phase to test for possible reactive foods.

Transitioning back to a more normal diet after you have finished your cleanse should be done in steps. Many people are reactive to common foods such as wheat, dairy, soy, sugar, peanuts, corn, and eggs—the Sensitive Seven. Wait for a while before you reintroduce these. Later you can retest those foods to see if they weaken your health. Add them one at a time, every day or two.

A brief review of the Sensitive Seven Elimination Diet, described in *The False Fat Diet*, will give you the general idea.

SAMPLE MENU: HYPOALLERGENIC DIET

DAY 1

Breakfast:
- Hot Breakfast Quinoa (page 225) or Gluten-Free Oatmeal (page 224) with 1 to 2 teaspoons honey (or maple syrup) and 2 tablespoons rice milk (4- to 6-ounce bowl)
- Fruit salad (6-ounce bowl with banana, apple, raisins)
- Hot herbal tea

Snack:
- Rice crackers or rice bread with 1 tablespoon almond butter or 1 tablespoon all-fruit spread
- Fruit juice (8-ounce glass)

Lunch:
- Tuna salad with sliced celery or onion and 1 to 2 tablespoons vinaigrette dressing
- Steamed and seasoned green beans (½ cup)
- Spelt or rice bread (1 slice) with 1 teaspoon almond butter or fruit spread

Snack:
- Carrot and celery sticks (5 to 10)
- Almonds (5 to 10) or sunflower seeds (20 to 40 or 1 handful)

Dinner:
- Stuffed Bell Peppers (page 228) or Herbed Soup (page 231) (12-ounce bowl)
- Green salad with 1 tablespoon vinaigrette dressing
- Iced herbal tea

Snack:
- Pears in Black Cherry Sauce (page 241) or 1 piece of fruit

DAY 2

Breakfast:
- Hot Breakfast Quinoa (page 225) and Baked Apples (page 225)
- Hot herbal tea

Snack:
- Apple
- Walnuts

Lunch:
- Gazpacho (page 231) and Green Pea Hummus (page 229)
- Iced herbal tea

Snack:
- Rice crackers

Dinner:
- Vegetable Curry (page 230) or Lentil Stew (page 230)
- Steamed broccoli
- Green salad with Ginger Garlic Dressing (page 236)

Snack:
- Baked Apples (page 225) with cinnamon raisins and 1 teaspoon honey

This eating plan is one of the most popular with patients because they usually feel better and lose weight. If you sense that you are reactive to foods other than the Sensitive Seven, such as tomatoes, potatoes, or oranges, you might want to eliminate them as well. In addition, you should eliminate any food you have been eating most every day or foods that you crave.

Your loss of water weight and adipose tissue in this eating plan will depend upon several factors. Among the most important is your activity level. If you are very active and exercise an hour or more each day, you may lose several pounds a week. If you are moderately active and exercise every other day, you may lose a pound or two each week. If you are inactive and don't exercise at all, you may not lose weight at all and might even gradually gain some weight. In addition, men will tend to lose adipose tissue on this eating plan more quickly than women, because men generally have a higher percentage of muscle and usually burn fat more efficiently.

Another factor that will determine your rate of weight loss is your size. Both men and women lose weight more quickly the more overweight they are. No, that isn't an excuse to gain more weight! If you are a very heavy person, you will tend to lose more weight on this eating plan than a small, lighter person. If you are inactive, or if you are a woman, you may need to eat somewhat less food than this eating plan calls for, in order to lose weight. You can do this by reducing your portion sizes or avoiding some of the foods the plan calls for.

After at least one week on this eating program, you may begin to reintroduce suspected reactive foods as you begin your food "challenges." You could also add pureed vegetable soups or a "cream" of vegetable soup blended with a very loose oatmeal instead of dairy. Another idea is to eat a lighter lunch or dinner on some days or just drink juice at those times.

The Detox Doc's Anti-Candida Diet

If you have been diagnosed with "Candida" or other yeast overgrowth, you will want to continue to avoid simple sugars (and alcohol and vinegars) even after you transition back to a long-term program. Avoid sugar, refined flours, and excessive use of natural sweeteners such as honey, maple syrup, fruit juice, turbinado sugar, and so forth. The bulk of your diet should be composed of vegetables, beans, peas, lentils, fish, nuts and seeds, olive oil, and to a lesser degree whole grains and high-quality meats. I usually have people limit fruit intake to one or two pieces and usually not overly sweet ones like melons. Berries are good and some apple or pear.

The overall approach to treating the yeast problem is threefold. The first facet is to refrain from feeding those "yeastie beasties" what they like to eat, so they can't thrive and divide. They live on mostly simple sugars, yeast, and fermented foods. These include fruits, fruit juices, and dried fruits, sugary foods, refined flour products, alcoholic beverages, cheese, vinegar, breads, and other yeasted fermented food products, such as soy sauce. All these foods are avoided on the anti-yeast diet except for occasional fruit if tolerated, as I just mentioned.

What to eat? There are many recommended foods—fish, poultry, meat, lots of vegetables, some whole grains, nuts, seeds, and occasional eggs. (The anti-yeast diet is more difficult for vegetarians, but definitely possible.) Some yogurt, especially acidophilus culture, is all right if milk is tolerated. Oils are obtained from the nuts and seeds, as well as from some butter and more cold-pressed vegetable oils, such as olive, flaxseed, sesame, and sunflower. Legumes are often limited because they add to intestinal gas. Initially, the diet includes no fruit, or only one piece a day, and none of the sweeter fruits, such as grapes, bananas, and melons.

Basic meals include proteins and vegetables or, occasionally, starch and vegetables. For the first few weeks, the starches and carbohydrates, including pastas and especially breads, are limited to one or two portions daily, mainly as whole-grain cereals. This includes some brown rice, millet, oatmeal, or corn polenta. Reducing starchy foods does lower the fiber intake, but usually other aspects of the treatment help colon function.

ANTI-YEAST DIET PLAN

Emphasize
- Vegetables (all beans)
- Meats*
- Nuts and seeds
- Poultry*
- Butter
- Eggs
- Cold-pressed oils
- Fish*
- Lemon
- Whole grains
- Fresh fruit**

Avoid
- Sugar (all forms)
- Baked goods
- Alcoholic beverages
- Vinegars
- Fruit juices
- Pickled vegetables
- Dried fruits
- Cheese
- Refined flours
- Mushrooms
- Breads

* Vegetarians will need to use more whole grains, beans, nuts, and seeds, but this higher carbohydrate diet does not really curb yeast as effectively. Furthermore, vegetarians seem to be more prone to yeast overgrowth because their diet is more alkaline and sweet, which supports the yeast. Yeast does not grow as well in an acid environment, and thus many of the anti-yeast herbs and medicines are fairly acidic.

** Limit to two pieces daily.

SAMPLE MENU: AFTER-DETOX DIET

Day 1

Fruit and/or juice:	Organic apple or Energizing Elixir juice (page 248)
Breakfast:	Hot Breakfast Quinoa (page 225)
Lunch:	White Bean Salad (page 233) and Fresh Harvest juice (page 249)
Snack:	Cold Almonds (page 239)
Dinner:	Salmon with Roasted Garlic and Rosemary (page 229)
Treat:	Juice Jells (page 240)

Day 2

Fruit and/or juice:	Organic grapes or Sunset Soother juice (page 249)
Breakfast:	Baked Apples (page 225)
Lunch:	Herbed Soup (page 231)
Snack:	Green Pea Hummus (page 229)
Dinner:	Kombu-Squash Soup (page 232)
Treat:	Fresh fruit juice or smoothie of your choice

Day 3

Fruit:	Grapefruit or After Workout Refresher juice (page 248)
Breakfast:	Basic Steel-Cut Oatmeal (page 224)
Lunch:	Jicama Salad (page 233) and Gazpacho (page 231)
Snack:	Kombu Knots (page 240)
Dinner:	Glazed Broccoli (page 233) and Lentil Stew (page 230)
Treat:	Pears in Black Cherry Sauce (page 241)

The anti-yeast diet can also be used to reduce yeast and parasites. This diet is a special therapeutic eating plan, and not necessarily a lifelong one, although many people like the way they feel on it. Intestinal symptoms decrease, energy improves, and itchy or irritated skin may start to heal with a decrease in sugar and yeasty foods. Also, some weight can be shed easily on this diet. This may be a problem for the already trim person, and lighter people need to emphasize regular eating to prevent weight loss, including more nuts and seeds and nut butters especially.

After a few weeks, we can test ourselves with fruit, bread, other grain products, or cheese—of course, one food at a time, and only one new one daily—to see how we handle them. If they seem to cause no problems, we can then bring these foods

Day 4

Fruit:	Cantaloupe or Tobin's Strawberry Almond Shake (page 245)
Breakfast:	Dr. Elson's Breakfast Rice (page 226)
Lunch:	Quick Southwest Quinoa (page 228)
Snack:	Fresh juice or smoothie of your choice
Dinner:	Vegetable Curry (page 230) with Date and Orange Chutney (page 237)
Treat:	Baked Apples (page 225)

Day 5

Fruit:	Purple Papaya smoothie (page 244)
Breakfast:	Breakfast Millet (page 225) or Baked Apples (page 225)
Lunch:	Stuffed Bell Peppers (page 228) and green salad with Ginger Garlic Dressing (page 236)
Snack:	Asian Cucumber Salad (page 234) and Carrot Cocktail (page 248)
Dinner:	Broccoli Soup (page 232) and Caramelized Onion Quinoa (page 235)
Treat:	Cold Almonds (page 239) and Cinnamon Cider (page 242)

Day 6

Fruit:	Pears and Apple Lemon Spritzer (page 243)
Breakfast:	Dani's Muesli (page 226)
Lunch:	Herbed Millet with Steamed Vegetables (page 228)
Snack:	Guacamole (page 240) with baby carrots
Dinner:	Caraway Cabbage Borscht (page 232)
Treat:	Gingered Green Tea (page 242) or Banana Soother smoothie (page 245)

into our diet on a rotating basis, like every few days. Eventually, adding more whole grains and fiber will provide what I believe is a healthier diet. Different degrees of strictness with the diet may be necessary, depending on the severity of the problem and the individual.

A more stringent diet might exclude all fruits; whole grains, particularly the glutinous ones—wheat, barley, rye, and oats; herb teas and spices, which may contain molds; and many nuts, which can also carry molds.

Other facets of a good anti-yeast program involve intake of healthy bacteria and probiotics, such as *Lactobacillus acidophilus* and Bifidobacteria. These help reduce yeast growth and provide what your colon wants. Also, take herbs and medicines that help kill or inhibit the yeast growth. These include such natural supplements as garlic, grapefruit seed extract, oregano oil, plant tannins, caprylic acid, undecylenic acid, and berberine (a goldenseal herb extract). Most of these substances can be a little irritating.

If garlic is used, take two capsules several times daily. Pau d'arco, a Brazilian tree bark, and other plant tannins are popular herbs in the treatment of yeast, allergies, and other immune problems. They can be taken in capsules, or tea made from the bark can be drunk several times daily. It seems to tone or strengthen the gastrointestinal tract and may help reduce yeast. Caprylic acid is popular; however, in sensitivity tests it doesn't appear to be very effective in eradicating the yeast. I often use short courses of systemic drugs to really clear candida and other yeasts. The most common one I prescribe is Nizoral (ketoconazole), and then Diflucan (fluconazole), and Sporanox (itraconoazale) and nystatin less commonly. Nystatin mainly helps lower intestinal yeast but is not absorbed and thus is not systemic like the other drugs mentioned, meaning they get into the bloodstream and are delivered to the tissues. The systemic drugs can cause some liver irritation, yet most people tolerate them well, and with stopping, the liver clears easily. I often have people use milk thistle (silymarin) herb, about 60 to 80 mg twice daily. Doing the whole program is the best way to clear candida-related problems. (Review chapter 17 in *Staying Healthy with Nutrition* for a more complete discussion.)

CHAPTER EIGHT

Teenagers and Detoxification

I WAS AN OVERWEIGHT TEENAGER MANY DECADES AGO as well as an overweight child and medical student. I ate the sweet and fatty American diet that came into place in the 1950s, and it kept me quite heavy. Due to my weight, my self-image and personal life were less than ideal. It wasn't until after finishing medical school and establishing my medical practice that I began to learn about what it takes to keep my body fit and vital. Yet, because of my early eating habits, I have struggles to this day to keep my weight down and my health up.

That is why I decided to add a new chapter for teenagers, to emphasize to you that the concepts and practices of health and detoxification are essential to learn and **begin as early as possible**. As a teenager, you are learning to take greater responsibility for your life. Your health is a crucial aspect of your life. It affects everything—the grades you earn, the sports you play and how good you are at playing them, the people you date, and the extracurricular activities you can participate in. Let me repeat that: Your health affects *everything*. My message to everyone, but especially to you young adults, is: **Lay the groundwork NOW for your future health. This begins with the choices you make every day. And I promise you; it matters now, and for a healthier future, too.**

Most of our habits begin when we're young, and most of the decisions we make about those habits are made casually—without much thought. In our early years, we usually feel the benefits more than the damage of our

---

DIET CHOICES: ROOM FOR IMPROVEMENT

Try and Enjoy:

Whole-grain products (examples: brown rice, oatmeal, quinoa)

Fresh fruits and vegetables

Roasted vegetables and potatoes

Poultry and fish

Water and fresh juices

Apples, raisins, and dates

Milk alternatives: rice, almond, or hemp

Avoid or Reduce:

Refined flour products (white rice and bread, noodles, cookies)

French fries and ketchup (fats, sugar, and calories)

Hamburgers

Soda

Candy and pastries

Cow's milk

Coffee

(Learn more about sugars in chapter 10.)

---

choices, such as the energy rush from sugar and caffeine, the easy highs from drinking alcohol, and the calming effects of tobacco. That's partly why some of these substances are illegal to use until eighteen or twenty-one years of age. Many of them are addictive, and trying to eliminate them later in life, when they begin to undermine our health, can be very challenging. This book is a guide to help disengage and detoxify from these common **SNACC habits—Sugar, Nicotine, Alcohol, Caffeine, and Chemicals.**

Most of our habits are already well established by (and during) our adolescent years. They are influenced by our parents, our communities, and our school environments. Our personal tastes are also shaped by the media and peer pressure. From ages eleven to seventeen (depending on when adolescence begins for you), it

is the time for enhanced growth. During these years our bodies need more nutrients than at almost any other time, other than pregnancy. This is the time when teens experience growth spurts, which can add 3 to 4 inches in height and 15 to 30 pounds in weight seemingly overnight but often yearly.

This is *not* the time to live solely on the "white food" diet—bread, cheese, sugar, pizza, pasta, and fries. We need a variety of foods in a variety of colors! Yes, that's those fruits and vegetables that can be so tasty and nourishing. Here, the concept of cellular health (see chapter 2) as the basis for overall good health becomes crystal clear: when our cells are healthy, guess what? So are we. When our cells are malnourished or stressed or polluted, we might get sick, gain weight, break out, or do poorly on a test. Our bodies' trillions of cells require vitamins, minerals, amino acids, fatty acids, and phytonutrients*— pretty scarce in candy, sodas, and gum—to keep us going every day. Toxins found in the air, water, and food also interfere with cell function. But healthy bodies do not get sick very easily because healthy cells can stand up to most invaders.

Phytonutrients include a wide variety of substances that support the body and give plants their color, flavor, and aroma.

A SAMPLING OF TEEN-FRIENDLY RECIPES

(See more recipes in part 3)

Cherry Ice

SERVES 1

1 cup frozen pitted dark cherries

1 cup ice

1 cup water

1 tablespoon cherry juice concentrate

1 teaspoon xylitol or Just Like Sugar (see page 135)

Combine all the ingredients in a blender, and blend as much or as little as desired.

Add sparkling mineral water for a bubbly kick and 1 teaspoon lemon juice for a hint of tartness, or you could use some honey or agave for more sweetness, too (optional).

Tropical Detoxifier

SERVES 2

1 cup pineapple juice

1 cup apple juice

1 cup ice

1 teaspoon grated fresh ginger

1 tablespoon freshly squeezed lemon juice

Combine all the ingredients in a blender and blend until smooth. Drink immediately.

Chai Cocoa

SERVES 1

1 cup rice milk

1 teaspoon dark unsweetened cocoa powder

1 teaspoon xylitol or Just Like Sugar (see page 135)

Pinch of cinnamon

Pinch of cardamom

1/4 teaspoon vanilla extract

In a small saucepan, combine all the ingredients over medium heat. Do not boil. Serve hot.

Oatmeal with Almonds and Fruit

SERVES 2

2 cups water
Pinch of salt
1 cup rolled oats

Toppings:
1 cup rice milk or almond milk
1 to 2 tablespoons maple syrup
2 tablespoons chopped toasted almonds
1/2 cup sliced strawberries and/or
   1/2 banana, sliced

Bring the water and salt to a boil in a pot and then stir in the rolled oats. Reduce the heat and let simmer for 15 to 18 minutes, stirring occasionally. Serve with nondairy milk, a drizzle of maple syrup, nuts, and fresh fruit.

Greek Yogurt with Fruit and Nuts

Greek yogurt has become increasingly popular thanks to its ultra-creamy texture. It's available in delicious flavors, including honey, vanilla, and exotic berry flavors such as acai and pomegranate. This is a healthy, quick breakfast solution loaded with nutrients. SERVES 1 TO 2

8 ounces Greek yogurt (plain or flavored)
1 piece of fruit, chopped (apple, plum, banana, peach)
2 to 3 tablespoons toasted chopped nuts (almonds, pecans, hazelnuts)

Combine all the ingredients in a bowl and devour!

Herbed Sweet Potato Fries

SERVES 2

1/4 cup extra virgin olive oil
3 cloves garlic, minced
2 large sweet potatoes
3 tablespoons fresh chopped rosemary
2 teaspoons salt
Black pepper to taste (or red pepper for a spicy version)

Preheat the oven to 350°F. Combine the olive oil and garlic in a large bowl. Slice the sweet potatoes into long strips. Add the potatoes to the olive oil and toss until each fry is well coated. Add the rosemary and salt and toss until each fry is well coated. Sprinkle with black pepper. Spread the fries onto a baking sheet and bake for 15 minutes. After 15 minutes, check the fries, turning them to ensure even browning, and continue cooking for another 10 to 15 minutes, until golden brown. Serve with ketchup or vegetable dip. If sweet potatoes are hard to find, you can substitute with russet or any variety of white potato for real home fries.

Island Coleslaw

SERVES 4

2 cups shredded cabbage

1 cup grated carrot

1 (8-ounce) can crushed pineapple, drained

1/4 cup rice vinegar

1/2 teaspoon caraway seeds

Pinch of black or red pepper

Salt to taste

Combine all the ingredients in a large bowl and mix well. Chill for at least an hour before serving.

Cilantro Guacamole

SERVES 2

1 large avocado

1/2 cup plain low-fat yogurt (optional)

1/4 cup fresh cilantro

1/4 to 1 teaspoon hot sauce (your preference)

2 cloves garlic

1 teaspoon lime juice

1/2 teaspoon salt

1/2 teaspoon black pepper or 1/4 teaspoon red pepper

Combine all the ingredients in a food processor, puree, and serve with baked rice chips or raw fresh vegetables for dipping. Or serve as a topping over rice chips, black beans, and jalapeños.

"HEALTHIER" FAST FOOD— REALITY OR OXYMORON?

Teens are typically very busy people. You're on the run to school, sports activities, and endless social events. It's no wonder you (and often your parents) choose fast food as a convenient meal. But teen obesity is on the rise—40 percent of American teens have been told by their doctors that they need to lose weight. That's nearly half the teenage population! Restaurant meals are usually higher in calories, saturated fat, sugar, and salt than a meal prepared at home. And fast food is notorious for staggeringly high calories, sugar, sodium, and unhealthy fats. A typical fast food meal often contains an entire day's worth of recommended calories and a week's worth of unhealthy fats. Recently, fast food chains have come under fire for their high-calorie menus and many are attempting to provide better choices.

The Big Breakfast with Hotcakes at McDonald's contains 56 grams of fat. The American Heart Association recommends we consume less than 60 grams of fat per day. So that's almost an entire day's worth of fat all in just one meal, and not the healthier fats either.

By being conscious of some of the typical fast food "traps," we can navigate their menus and stay healthy! A good way to start is to make a list of what you consider special treat foods—fries, potato chips, pastries, cookies, candy, pizza, burgers, sodas, shakes—and think about them as a small portion of your healthy diet.

FAST FOOD PITFALLS AND TIPS

Go online before you dine
It can be overwhelming when friends are waiting for you, your stomach is growling, and you're thinking about how much (or how little) cash you have for your meal. So decide what you're going to order before you even leave the house. This really lowers the stress of eating out and helps you stay on track. Visit www.healthydining finder.com.

Be aware of description seduction
Don't be duped by fancy culinary terms that mask the fatty, high-calorie reality. "Scalloped" means baked with milk and probably butter, "alfredo" means a butter- and cream-based sauce, "au gratin" means made with cheese and butter, and "basted" means that melted fat was poured over it.

Avoid fat-soaked foods
To lower fat and calorie intake, avoid anything deep-fried, pan-fried, batter-dipped, breaded, creamy, or crispy. These are simply different ways to say dipped in or enhanced with fat.

Avoid "empty" liquid calories
Sodas, slushies, milkshakes, lemonade, and many fruit juices are loaded with sugar, are surprisingly high in calories, and contain virtually nothing nutritious.

Drink water
We need water to keep our skin clear, move our bowels, and boost our energy. Plus it's free—and filling.

Review the menu
Most fast food establishments now post nutritional information, such as calories and fats, for each item they serve.

LEVELS OF DETOXING FOR TEENS

The term "detoxing" describes a process that eliminates certain foods from your diet for a limited, defined period of time. Detoxing can be as simple as taking a break from sugar for a few weeks, or it can be a lengthier, more involved program, such as juice cleansing. We would like here to offer four levels of detoxing for teenagers.

Level 1: Breaking or Changing a Habit

At any age, once a habit has become, well, a habit, it will be a challenge to change. Popular wisdom has it that it takes three weeks to establish a new routine and three months to truly break a habit. It also takes desire and a sensible, workable plan. And for some of us, it takes a crisis (health, relationship, financial) to motivate a change.

Let moderation be your guide

We can get by with eating just about anything once in a while, but having your special treat foods more than two to three times a week may be too much. French fries, anyone? Not as your primary vegetable, please.

Skip "dressing" disasters

Be aware of those über-high-calorie dressings such as creamy salad dressings, sour cream, creamy spreads, and mayonnaise-based dipping sauces. Use them minimally, or try a vinaigrette instead.

Special order

Exercise your right to modify; ask for dressing on the side so you can use as little as you'd like, order sandwiches without the mayo-based dressings, order potatoes with the butter and sour cream on the side, and ask for vegetables steamed, not cooked in oil or butter.

Control portion sizes

Portion sizes are so big now that it's easy to lose sense of what a normal serving looks like. Order the small size, knowing you can always order more if you're still hungry. If you order a full meal, eat half, and take the rest home for another meal.

Focus on your food

Try to relax while you're eating. Avoid eating on the run or while driving or watching TV. Distractions can keep you from realizing when you're full.

Visualize a healthy meal

A healthy meal is hard to find at a fast food restaurant, but there are better options. The chart on pages 108 and 109 offers the best menu options at several fast food restaurants.

Usually, the younger we are, the easier it is to change; yet, this is not always the case. Motivation is important to success, as is support from family and friends. If you try to stop smoking or drinking, but you still want to hang out with your smoking and drinking friends, you will find it very difficult—tortuous, in fact. Why hassle yourself in that way?

My sixteen-year-old patient Jan had a group of girlfriends who were experimenting with drugs that included alcohol, marijuana, and amphetamines. They began cutting school and getting into trouble, which resulted in an ultimatum from Jan's parents. Jan got some counseling and was able to change her activities—and her friends. She made the soccer team and started seeing a boy who did not do drugs— which meant she had a lot less time for her girlfriends. Jan set herself up for success.

BEST AND WORST FAST-FOOD CHOICES

We have reviewed a few popular fast-food menus and found the following choices—based on calories, fats, and sugars—to be healthier options when this book went to press. We already know these are not the highest quality foods, but we understand that value for money is certainly a factor. We hope more healthy options will be available in the future. Even the basic burger, fries, and soda have loads of calories from fats and sugars without much nutrition, although the beef patty has some protein, as does the cheese (with some calcium). Realize that eating fast foods from the restaurants listed here ideally should be an occasional "treat" and not your regular fare. Whenever possible, avoid high-fat, processed meats like pepperoni.

McDonald's

Best	Premium Caesar Salad with Grilled Chicken	190 calories
	Chicken McNuggets 4 piece	190 calories
	McCafé Wild Berry Real Fruit Smoothie (12 oz.)	210 calories
	McCafé Iced Nonfat Latte (small)	50 calories
	Fruit and Maple Oatmeal without brown sugar	290 calories
Worst	Angus Chipotle BBQ Bacon	800 calories
	Frappe Mocha (large)	680 calories
	McCafé Chocolate Shake (22 oz.)	880 calories
	Big Breakfast with Hotcakes (large biscuit)	1,150 calories

Burger King

Best	Tender Grill Garden Salad	230 calories
	1% Chocolate Lowfat Milk	180 calories
	Fruit Topped Maple Flavor Quaker Oatmeal	270 calories
	Seattle's Best Coffee Regular (black, medium)*	0 calories
Worst	Triple Whopper	1,140 calories
	Double Croissant'wich with Double Sausage	700 calories
	BK Ultimate Breakfast Platter	1,310 calories
	Oreo BK Sundae Chocolate Shake (medium)	920 calories

* With 1 tablespoon milk and 1 teaspoon sugar, add 34 calories

Arby's

Best	Eggs Scrambled (breakfast)	70 calories
	Light Grilled Chicken Salad	280 calories
	Iced Tea (no sugar)	0 calories
Worst	Philly Chicken Baked Potato	880 calories
	Italian Sub	800 calories
	Chocolate Shake (regular)	570 calories

Carl's Jr.

Best	Kids Hamburger	280 calories
	Cranberry, Apple, Walnut Grilled Chicken Salad	360 calories
	Original Grilled Chicken Salad (without dressing)	270 calories
Worst	The Western Bacon Six Dollar Burger	1,030 calories
	Loaded Breakfast Burrito	780 calories
	Big Country Breakfast Burrito	750 calories

KFC

Best	Chicken Breast without breading or skin	160 calories
	KFC Snacker, Honey BBQ	210 calories
	Grilled Drumstick Value Box	380 calories
Worst	Crispy Twister	610 calories
	Chicken Pot Pie	790 calories
	KFC Famous Bowls Mashed Potato and Gravy	680 calories

Domino's

Best	Pacific Veggie Pizza (1 slice)	245 calories
	Thin-Crust Pepperoni Pizza (1 slice)	170 calories
	Hawaiian Pizza (1 slice)	90 calories
	Veg-A-Roma (1 slice)	139 calories
Worst	Chicken Parm Sandwich	766 calories
	Philly Cheese Steak Pizza (1 slice)	260 calories
	Cheesy Bread (1 piece)	930 calories

Change requires a sensible, achievable plan, as Jan's story demonstrates. Whenever we decide to cut something out of our lives, we are making space for something new. Filling those spaces with better replacements is key.

Level 2: Elimination Diets

Is it hard for you to drag yourself out of bed in the morning? Do you have acne or weird skin rashes? What about digestive upset, constipation, or flatulence (and smelly farts)? Are you gaining weight in the wrong places? All of these issues can come from our diet choices, which is why a temporary elimination diet is a good way to test what agrees with us and what doesn't. In fact, taking a break from certain foods is often the *only* way to make the connection that they aren't doing us any good.

To begin an elimination diet, choose some key foods (or substances, if this applies to you) that you feel most attached to. For my adult patients, I suggest they begin with the key **five foods/substances: wheat, dairy, sugar, caffeine, and alcohol.** Some patients volunteer to also avoid red meat and fried foods, but you can start by eliminating just one food or one group of foods. (Or, start by eliminating more foods, then even after just a week or two, gradually reinstate them as a test.) As you begin to feel—and look—better, you can try eliminating a few more items. For example, if you have problems with acne outbreaks, do a personal meal inventory—and be honest! If fried foods, dairy products, and baked goods rank high on the list (meaning

CASE STUDY: B.B., AGE 19

B.B. went to Daniella looking for ways to counter the negative effects of her daily cigarette smoking. She made it clear that she did not intend to stop smoking entirely, but she'd made the decision to cut back. Daniella recommended following each cigarette with a 500 mg chewable vitamin C to help reduce the free radicals (potentially damaging molecules) produced in her body from smoking. B.B. decided to reduce her smoking from twenty to ten cigarettes a day, and to smoke half a cigarette at a time. When asked why she didn't plan to quit, she said she'd miss her smoking breaks at work, which her nonsmoking coworkers didn't get. This realization eventually spurred her to seek some emotional cleansing from a mind-body therapist to help her quit smoking.

French fries and/or pizza are included in three or more meals a week) consider avoiding them for three weeks. That means, hold the fries (and the potato chips, while you're at it) and replace the pizza and shake with a big mixed-veggie and protein salad and iced tea for three weeks, and see what happens. If you start getting comments on your complexion and smaller jean size, you may want to move on to the next level.

The way to test the foods you eliminated is to bring them back slowly, one at a time every two days, and pay attention to how you feel. Do you notice any symptoms returning that had cleared during the elimination? Observe any physical, mental, or mood changes within an hour or so of consuming the food, then observe again several hours later, and observe again the following morning when you awaken. If you have noticeable reactions, you may wish to avoid that food or substance for a longer period.

Level 3: The Detox Diet with a Little Added Protein

The Detox Diet focusing on vegetables with some fruit and grains makes it a bit easier to follow a specifically targeted elimination diet and healing program, helping the body become trimmer (better-fitting jeans) and more energetic, often with reduced cravings. The initial eating plan is fruit and grains in the morning along with vegetables and protein at lunch and dinner. The protein can be some fish, poultry, or meat, or for vegetarians, it can be beans. When you focus on what you are eating at breakfast, lunch, and dinner, you will become less concerned about the things you are *not* eating.

If you are ready to try the Detox Diet for a week or two or three, follow the guidance in chapter 5. I recommend taking a few supplements during this program as well. These might include a multiple vitamin-mineral, some green algae powder, vitamin C, and some alkaline minerals, such as potassium, magnesium, and calcium. It's also wise to add calcium when you are avoiding milk products either temporarily or long term.

Level 4: Juice Cleansing, a Possibility

A juice-cleansing program means that only juices are consumed for a limited, clearly defined period of time. It is a more extreme program, but definitely doable by teenagers. But you must be monitored carefully, and a lower-calorie, lower-nutrient short-term experience must be appropriate for you, which means you must be in a reasonably good state of health to begin with. I've had many teens in my detox and cleansing groups over the years, and I haven't lost any yet! In fact, they tend to do quite well—often with even more striking results than the adults—their nasal congestion disappears, they wake up more easily, they do better on tests, and their clothes fit better. Many report having more confidence and feeling more in charge of their lives.

For anyone doing a cleansing program, it's essential to listen to your body and adapt as needed. Sometimes that means drinking some warm broth because you feel cold; at other times, you may need more protein because of fatigue. **If you decide you want to try a juice cleanse, be sure to inform your parents.** (Also, review chapter 4 for a more complete understanding and guidelines for healthy juice cleansing.)

NUTRIENT SUPPORT FOR TEENS

No one should start a detox program, at any level, without some additional nutrient support. This is especially crucial for anyone under the age of twenty-one. I recommend a basic multiple vitamin-mineral formula to ensure basic levels of all required nutrients. To support healthy skin and immune function, add **vitamin A** (about 5,000 to 10,000 IUs per day) and **zinc** (15 to 30 mg); **vitamin C** powder with extra minerals, especially **calcium, magnesium, and potassium** for healthy cell growth; and **green powders,** such as **chlorella** and **barley grass** to support the cleansing process.

TEEN HEALTH ISSUES

Acne and Skin Health

Acne is a common problem that results from (normal) hormonal changes, as well as food choices and skin cleanliness. In some cases, it is the result of oily, plugged hair follicles especially on the face, neck, and back. Acne can be mild or moderate in the form of blackheads, whiteheads, or small inflamed bumps. The more severe cystic acne can be quite painful and may leave scars.[1] I believe we heal the skin from the inside out, and this means our diet is very important. The all-American diet of childhood is rich in high-fat dairy foods frequently containing hormones (cow's milk, cheese, ice cream) and high

in sugar (cereals, sweets, snack foods, soda).[2] In my practice, I've noticed that a diet high in fried oils and trans fats (chips and fries—sorry) seems to be a frequent contributor to acne outbreaks and skin eruptions. So when treating patients with skin problems, I usually start improving their fat intake by prescribing healthier vegetable and fish oils. Also, dairy products seem to be linked to acne problems more than many other foods.

Balancing hormones is a bit more challenging. As a general rule, boys have more trouble with acne than girls do, and testosterone is often the culprit. However, dietary and detoxification measures can help, including avoiding foods that are high in refined sugar, dairy, fried foods, and bread.

CASE STUDY: M.L., AGE 18

M.L. went to Daniella seeking nutritional guidance for acne and depression. His diet was basically healthy, but he admitted to smoking marijuana to help relieve depression and anxiety. With Daniella's help, he realized his eating patterns changed radically after every joint. Instead of fresh fruit, big salads, and lean protein, he craved (and consumed) potato chips, ice cream, and candy washed down with quarts of soda. Once he made the connection, he stopped smoking pot, the cravings never returned, and his acne cleared up—which was a huge boost to his self-confidence.

Weight Problems

Most everyone thinks he or she is fat. And in truth, the media inform us that nearly two-thirds of Americans are overweight or obese. If you are overweight, this book can help you achieve a healthier weight naturally. I have found through my practice that weight loss comes easiest when we focus on eating healthfully for life rather than for a limited period of time. This means focusing on good-quality foods—meaning higher in nutrition and lower in calories and fats—on a daily basis.

Let this new way of eating be a positive influence on your family and friends. Be a leader of your own health and an inspiration to others. There are many extreme diets out there, like the popular high-protein (and high-fat), no-carb diets that severely restrict the variety of other foods that make up a balanced diet. Raw food and rigid vegetarian diets, while seemingly healthy, can cause deficiency problems if not used with some flexibility. (My personal philosophy is that if something sounds too extreme—it probably is!) Of course, there are weight-loss programs that focus on vegetables and protein, reducing carbohydrates, and totally avoiding sugars and junk foods. For many people, this may be a sensible approach to moderate weight loss and stable weight maintenance. But I believe the key to long-term health is a diet that's well balanced with a wide variety of whole, nutritious foods. Overall, the Detox Diet and the

Daniella's Demise

When I was in ninth grade, I decided I wanted to lose some weight and went with the then-popular salad bar strategy. When friends and I went out for lunch, I always opted for the salad bar. I thought everything at the salad bar was healthy and it seemed the perfect way to get more vegetables into my diet. I ate huge servings smothered in ranch dressing, bacon bits, nuts, and olives. Boy was I wrong! I gained about 8 pounds in two months. I was stressed out about not fitting into the new clothes I'd saved up for all summer, and the worst part for me was that I gained all my weight in my thighs, hips, and butt. I was called Thunder Thighs, and the nickname stuck throughout high school. Fortunately, my best friend gently explained that I should consider switching to a lower-fat vinaigrette dressing and avoid the bacon and olives—which can have up to 40 calories *per piece*. It was an "aha!" moment for me. It took me months to lose the weight, but I did start asking for nutrition information for the foods that I was eating on a regular basis so I wouldn't be blindsided again.

programs found here are to help you transition to this healthier, lifelong eating program that nourishes you completely.

Eating Disorders: Anorexia and Bulimia

Some people develop severe problems with food, what we call *eating disorders* and are familiar to most as anorexia and bulimia. Eating disorders are a steadily growing health concern in the United States, especially for parents. Anorexia is diagnosed when the patient tries to avoid eating altogether and typically becomes dangerously thin; bulimia involves binge eating followed by purging, whether through self-induced vomiting or the abuse of laxatives. These disorders often affect teenagers like you. There are many schools of thought about the causes of these complex psychological conditions and their often tragic physiological consequences. **I do not recommend fasting or any extreme form of detoxing for young people with eating disorders. However, most people can benefit from following the healthy guidelines in this book, which includes eating three nourishing meals per day.** If you or someone you know is struggling with food challenges, it is imperative to get experienced professional help in the form of counseling. Attempting to resolve such issues on your own is potentially life threatening. Good intentions are simply not enough. Please get help.

Alcohol Use and Binge Drinking

Moderate consumption of alcohol is generally well tolerated by most people. However, like many things in life, when it's consumed to excess, it can be toxic—even lethal. We all know the legal drinking age in the United States is twenty-one. But we also know that when something is outlawed or off limits, it often becomes even more desirable. During our teen years, we are often testing limits, as is done with alcohol and other drugs. This also comes with a greater risk of accidents from fast and/or drunk driving. Teen time is also one for developing wisdom along with experience, and making wise choices are important at all times.

According to the 2010 National Survey on Drug Use and Health, more than 26 percent of American twelve- to twenty-year-olds report drinking alcohol.[3] And 23 percent of twelfth graders admit to binge drinking.[4] Many more drink occasionally or get drunk at parties with their friends.

It is well established that alcohol affects not only behavior but also brain development, and the brain is still developing during our teen years. Avoiding alcohol during these years will help create healthier adults. Studies have shown that consequences—both legal and parental—can deter teens from drinking excessively. But ultimately, our own good judgment is the key.

Many problems from drinking alcohol can occur, no matter what your age. Alcohol is a depressant of the nervous system and, perhaps surprisingly, a mood depressant—after an initial apparent lift. During our teen years, when the brain and nervous system are still growing and adapting, the effects of alcohol can be especially harmful. Alcohol is also hard on the liver and other organs. (You can read more about the physiological risks of alcohol in chapter 12.) It never hurts to be wise and moderate at any age.

When we are young, we can have both a sensitive nervous system and emotional makeup, and we also may be more able to handle toxins in the form of alcohol with our resilient, healthy bodies. We all know that alcohol intoxication can cause auto accidents and fatalities. For these and other reasons, our government and lawmakers have decided that people under 21 years of age cannot drink legally. Furthermore, no one of any age can drink and drive. Everyone knows that these days.

Drugs

Substance use and abuse is prevalent in all age groups in our society. Thus, education is vitally important for the wise use or avoidance of alcohol, nicotine, and other drugs. As a health-focused doctor, I can say, like all lifestyle habits, it matters what we do and how we do it, what we know and how we apply it, and everything we do contributes to our health outcome.

For a variety of reasons, teenagers (and adults) can have issues with drug abuse, be it marijuana, amphetamines, or the various psychedelics. This use and abuse can be both the result of and the cause

CASE STUDY: R.M., AGE 13

R.M. was tall for his age, with an athletic build. But he felt tired and depressed, complained of chronic headaches, and had little interest in food—except carbohydrates. His diet diary revealed a daily intake of 4 to 5 liters of cola! Daniella suspected the sugar in the soda was filling him up, which affected his appetite, and the caffeine in the cola was the cause of the headaches. Not only that, but although he was drinking soda throughout the day and evening, he was actually *dehydrated*. Daniella recommended a schedule for cutting back on the soda to half the amount each day until it was entirely eliminated. So, on day one his intake was 2 liters, on day two it was 1 liter, on day three it was 1/2 liter and so on. The gradual elimination over the course of a week helped reduce the severity of the headaches (due to the withdrawal from the caffeine). The soda was replaced with a flavored effervescent vitamin powder made by Alacer called Emergen-C. R.M.'s favorites were the Apricot-Mango, Cherry-Pomegranate, and Orange-Pineapple Explosion. Incidentally, his weight dropped from 210 pounds to a healthier 186 over the following 12 weeks.

of emotional imbalance, depression and anxiety, and behavior issues. It can also affect your psychological well-being for the future. As with alcohol and cigarettes, education is helpful, as is counseling to help you cope with life's stresses and challenges.

TEN TIPS FOR TEENS

These are your **growth years** (mainly ages 13 to 16)—adding inches and pounds—and thus, your nutritional needs are great. I often tell teen patients that their nutrient needs are similar to those of a pregnant woman growing a baby, in regard to the additional protein, iron, calcium, and other nutrients required, and the need to avoid toxins that can injure cells, stunt growth, and weaken overall health.

1. **Eat nutritionally rich foods**—these are natural foods with vitamins; minerals; amino acids from proteins; fatty acids from nuts, seeds, and oils; and phytonutrients from fresh fruits and vegetables.

2. **Create a balanced diet and menu plans,** for general good health, and especially if you are challenged with foods or weight. Balance means a variety of nutritious foods, not just the same foods all the time. Balance also means wholesomeness, with a focus on fresh foods rather than packaged and processed ones.

3. **Pay attention to SNACC habits.** If you consume excess Sugar, become dependent on Caffeine for energy, or Alcohol for social activities, take a break and gain some perspective and guidelines for using these psychoactive substances. Obviously, don't smoke. Nicotine is very addictive, so once you begin it's challenging to stop.

4. Clarify for yourself a list of **"treats" in your diet.** Are they sweets or fast foods, for example? Allowing these as occasional foods and not as the basis of your diet is a wise plan. Maybe 10 percent of your diet could be treat foods—these may be candy, cookies, chips, fries, and sodas. How much of your diet is made up of treats now, and what can you do to change that?

As a teenager, your future health begins now and is affected by everything you do. There are many hazards and pitfalls in our modern culture, and it is often too easy to engage in the activities of substance use and abuse, be it sugar, smoking, caffeine and stimulant use, alcohol intake, and other drugs. This chapter is provided to offer you some ideas and support for your health now and in the future. Enjoy yourselves and your lives; I encourage this. Also know that sometimes the little things we do daily contribute to the bigger problems we suffer later. Thus, I encourage all people, young to old, to practice preventive medicine and care for themselves as if their lives depended on it. And it does!

5. **Don't let your weight get out of hand.** Any excess weight added during your teen years becomes part of you and is challenging to release later without hard work. Plus, excess weight can lead to many problems in adulthood. If you are already overweight, take steps to rebalance through more intelligent food choices and exercise.

6. **Play sports and exercise regularly—**it's good for your body, your mind, and your social life. Make sure you stretch and stay fit. Regular exercise is also a great way to manage stress and to help cleanse the body. **Quality and sufficient sleep is also vitally important for health,** so don't give up your rest and recharge time for other activities.

7. **When leaving home for college or for other reasons,** plan to maintain some controls and a healthy weight. Moving away from home, the controls you need will be self-motivated. Write out some guidelines (your parents can even help with this, if you like) for living that will work for you.

8. **Keep your mind positive—**learn relaxation exercises and maintain a positive attitude toward life. Love yourself and claim, "This is the only body I have, and I am going to treat it with love."

9. **Look for positive influences** to support your health, especially if you do not have this currently in your own family. Who can you talk with who will listen, not judge, and offer healthful guidance? It could be your school counselor, aunt or uncle, neighbor, or sibling. This is especially important for emotional well-being.

10. Even though you may feel immortal now, life is finite. **How you live now—**the choices you make every day—determine your future health, vitality and longevity. Stay Healthy!

Endnotes

1. Dan Kern, "Types of Acne," Acne.org. www.acne.org/types-of-acne.html (accessed November 27, 2011); F.W. Danby, "Nutrition and Acne," *Clinical Dermatology* 28, no. 6 (Nov-Dec, 2010): 598–604.

2. B.B. Davidovici and R. Wolf, "The Role of Diet in Acne: Facts and Controversies," *Clinical Dermatology* 28, no. 1 (Jan-Feb 2010): 12–6.

3. The Century Council, "Underage Drinking Research," www.centurycouncil.org/learn-the-facts/underage-drinking-research (accessed November 27, 2011).

4. The Century Council, "Underage Alcohol Consumption," www.centurycouncil.org/underage-drinking/underage-alcohol consumption (accessed November 27, 2011).

CHAPTER NINE

Life Stages and Special Circumstances

AS WITH SEEKING THE MOST APPROPRIATE medical care, choosing the right detox program may be affected by age, gender, and individual health status and require different diets, menu plans, and supplements. In the previous chapter, we focused on the challenging time of adolescence, so you teenagers, refer to that chapter. In this chapter, we will take a brief look at other stages of life as well as specific health conditions that may require extra caution before considering a detox program.

CHILDREN

Ideally, children start their lives eating the cleanest, most wholesome food. It saddens me to see a five- or ten-year-old clutching a bag of chips or artificially colored candies or a can of cola, not realizing the hooks of caffeine and sugar and fat are already firmly embedded in their young bodies. I believe there is a connection between these kinds of so-called foods and nervous system overstimulation in children. Further, I believe early exposure to these foods could be a contributing factor to energy and mood disorders in children, such as ADHD (Attention Deficit Hyperactivity Disorder).

As most of us know, we have a childhood overweight and obesity epidemic in the United States—the direct result of our modern lifestyle of inactivity combined with high-calorie, high-fat food choices. Children require *balanced*, nourishing meals comprised of the freshest, highest-quality foods possible. Where food is concerned, parents *must* think preventively on behalf of their kids and be the best role models they can be! And if your child is having problems, like recurring ear infections or constant digestive upset, an elimination diet can be very helpful in detecting the cause or causes (cow's milk and wheat products are often the culprits). It's never too early to clean up habits like sugar and caffeine, even in very young children. Kids can even handle a modified Detox Diet if you add some healthy protein to the menu, such as fish, poultry, or beans, and make sure they get enough healthy oils. **And always consult your pediatrician before starting your child on any sort of regimen.**

You won't always be able to monitor what your kids eat, but preparing their school lunches and keeping your fridge full of healthy and delicious snacks will help keep them on the right track. Nutritional content appears on every packaged food label in the United States, which means every one of us can make informed decisions about what we buy for our families. Remember—and remind them—**it's more fun to be healthy than it is to be sick.**

MEN

Generally, men tolerate fasting better than women do—although they are far less likely to take on such a program! When they do, they usually lose more weight more quickly. I often say that the most difficult part of any detox plan or elimination diet is deciding to actually *do* it. That's why participating in a detox group is so helpful—group members keep one another motivated when things get challenging. However, many people successfully complete these programs on their own. For some of us, simply the *idea* of delaying the onset of common medical problems, such as cardiovascular diseases, arthritis, back pain, diabetes, and cancer is enough to keep us on track. For me, feeling youthful and healthy well into my mid-sixties has been its reward. I want that for you, too, gentlemen, and for all those that you care about. In short, I want you to Stay Healthy so you don't have to Get Healthy!

The detox process helps eliminate body fat and retained water, with the added benefit of reducing inflammation. This, in turn, seems to help reduce other conditions, such as elevated blood pressure and cholesterol levels—all too common among American men. In fact, I have seen, over the course of time, the need for blood pressure and cholesterol medications diminish in some of my male patients. Men are also rightly concerned about prostate and sexual health. I recommend adding good fats (mainly omega-3 oils), more zinc, and less iron to their diets. (Typically, men don't need iron unless they are having blood loss.) I also suggest more supplemental magnesium than calcium. (For most women, the opposite is true—they tend to need more calcium and iron during the childbearing years.)

In addition to advocating for a healthy relationship to food, I prescribe healthy relationships with family, friends, and colleagues to my male patients. The former may include taking the occasional holiday from SNACCs (see part 2) or any overused, unhealthy foods. This doesn't mean giving up all your favorite things, but it does mean examining your relationship to them. The latter (healthy relationships) requires honesty and communication, and being aware of how each activity or individual affects you. I believe your spouse or partner, parents or children, friends, neighbors, and coworkers will appreciate the effort.

WOMEN

My female patients tend to embrace the detox process, and most benefit physically, emotionally, and spiritually. However, women must guard against becoming nutritionally deficient by making sure they get enough iron, calcium, protein, and the essential fatty acids from olive and flaxseed oils. There are times when women should not detox, such as during pregnancy or when they're nursing. Other contraindications are mentioned below.

As a rule, most women should pay attention to their intake of refined sugar. Not only does it contribute to weight gain, but also sugar can affect the menstrual cycle. My female patients who give up sugar report less pain, irritability, and swelling during their periods. Salt intake also causes swelling and contributes to high blood pressure. Finding the correct balance of sugar and salt in the diet is an important consideration for everyone.

Ladies, your personal relationships are very important to your overall health and emotional well-being. Therefore, I encourage you to include your spouse or partner and other family members in whichever detox program you choose. Once they learn about and understand the significance of detoxification, you'll have an in-house cheering section! Maybe your partner will want to join you. Detoxing can be one of the best relationship-enhancing experiences available. I've had the professional and personal satisfaction of watching couples change as they've detoxed together.

The process seems to improve communication, deepen compassion, and energize couple dynamics.

We do not recommend fasting or juice cleansing during menses. However, menstruating women in good health can safely complete the Detox Diet and the Smoothie Cleanse. Add algae and protein powder to boost your energy. My female patients tell me drinking warm broths and vegetable soups is particularly comforting.

Pregnancy and Nursing

During these important times in a woman's (and baby's) life, it's essential to make good food choices. Overall, a balanced diet full of nutrient-rich, preferably organic fresh fruits and vegetables, whole grains and beans, nuts and seeds, fish and other lean protein make up the optimal plan. Enhance your diet with fresh juices and smoothies for easy-to-digest nourishment. Supplements, including iron, calcium, protein, zinc, and essential fatty acids, are extremely helpful during this nutritionally demanding time in a woman's life. **We do not recommend any intense detox programs during pregnancy or the first six months of breastfeeding, when the mother is typically the sole source of her child's nutrition.** Avoiding alcohol and nicotine during pregnancy and nursing are well-established ideas. Avoiding empty-but-high-calorie junk foods is also a good idea. The best time to eliminate potentially troublesome habits like caffeine and sugar use is before you become pregnant. You can review more on

all these topics in chapter 15 of *Staying Healthy with Nutrition*.

Menopause

Menopause is a challenging transition for some women. Many female patients have told me that a week or two of an elimination diet or detoxification program is very helpful in boosting energy, improving moodiness, regulating sleep patterns, and reducing the severity of some of the uncomfortable symptoms, such as hot flashes and weight gain. In fact, several patients have reported that the 10-day fast kick-started a long-term weight reduction goal, launched an overall change in diet, and even altered their mental outlook. In my experience, detoxing and fasting are safe for menopausal women as long as they are not underweight or suffering from any serious disease.

ELDERS

Both Daniella and I have seen many seniors in their sixties and seventies who have flourished in our detox groups. Generally speaking, advancing age is not a factor when it comes to cleansing the body and adopting a new diet plan. However, if you are underweight or chronically fatigued, it is wise to consult your physician before embarking on any new regimen. That said, using the Detox Diet with some added protein for a week or two can be a useful transition as you shift toward a healthier way of eating. And adding a smoothie once or twice a day is an easy way to maintain body weight as we age. If the problem is that too much food is stressing your body and causing discomfort, then an elimination diet, fast, or juice cleanse is an excellent way to get you back on track. Stay strong and light.

CONDITIONS AND DISEASES

Weight Loss and Low Weight
I believe periodic detoxification is a useful practice for nearly everyone; however, when we eat a limited diet, we are likely to lose weight. This usually is a welcome "side benefit" for most people. However, if you are underweight, or already a normal weight for your height and build, losing additional pounds may not be a good idea. You can still detox by adapting the program through the addition of high-calorie foods and eating more frequently. This may include adding smoothies and fresh vegetable juices between meals, as well as snacks that include nuts and seeds, and adding grains or beans to meals. If the calorie count stays similar to your usual diet, your weight should be maintained.

Fatigue, Anemia, and Hypothyroidism
I would certainly encourage those who have been diagnosed with any of these conditions to try an elimination diet (especially from wheat, dairy, corn, sugar, and soy) and a detox plan. **However, I do not recommend fasting or consuming a restrictive diet for very long,** because symptoms may get worse. The key here is to include other nourishing and caloric foods like nuts and seeds, grains and legumes, and lots of fresh vegetables. Some animal proteins may be helpful as well. As always, consult your physician or endocrinologist before starting a new diet.

Diabetes and Low Blood Sugar
Blood sugar issues can be well handled during detox and cleansing programs if people consume calories at least every two to three hours during the day, especially with low blood sugar issues. For people with diabetes, their caloric intake is typically less, so this can be helpful and they may need to work with a physician to lower their medicines, especially with any juice cleansing. Thus, with diabetes it is best not to do fasting with juices that are high in sugars, such as apple, orange, and carrot. With a higher fruit and vegetable diet, it's good to add some amino acids, protein powder, or blue-green algae, which are higher in nutrients and amino acids. I have had many patients with diabetes and low blood sugar do fine with detox programs because the calorie intake is lower than usual and the food choices are typically healthier. Other supplements can be used to balance the sugar issues, such as the blue-green algae just mentioned, as well as protein powders, the minerals chromium and vanadium, adrenal glandular, B vitamins, and vitamin C. Juice cleansing with diabetes needs to be done with caution (especially

with insulin dependence) and with an experienced medical guide.

Heart and Blood Vessel Disease

I believe that the detoxification process may help prevent, or at least delay, the incidence and progression of blood vessel atherosclerosis and subsequent heart disease.

Improving circulation, reducing high blood pressure, and minimizing arterial plaque are the keys to avoiding heart and stroke. Studies suggest that an alkaline, nutrient-rich diet that's high in fiber and vegetable foods, along with regular exercise, may help lower and maintain blood cholesterol levels as well as blood viscosity (thickness), thus lowering incidence of atherosclerosis, high blood pressure, and high cholesterol. For more information on cardiovascular disease prevention, see chapter 16 in *Staying Healthy with Nutrition*.

Cancer

The heart disease prevention plan outlined above may also help reduce our risks for certain kinds of cancer. In my opinion, the only sensible approach to cancer is to attempt its prevention. I believe lifestyle is the key to this prevention, and this begins with not smoking and avoiding toxic environmental and food chemicals as much as possible. A balanced, nutritious diet comprised of organic protein and produce can only be beneficial. It is now accepted in the mainstream medical community that stress is frequently a trigger to many serious health problems, thus avoiding

extreme physical and chronic emotional stress is advisable.

I believe the processes of detoxification as described in this book can help make our bodies run more smoothly and efficiently by reducing the toxic load they otherwise have to cope with. Therefore, it stands to reason that most of us will benefit from preventive results offered by periodic detoxing, even taking into account variations in individual health status and genetic makeup. That's my message, after thirty years as a healer—the best treatment is prevention. And it all starts with making better decisions about our nutrition.

However, if you or someone you love is diagnosed with some form of cancer, please discuss with your physician and oncologist the possible pros and cons of detoxification, especially following treatment.

Mercury and Metal Toxicity

Mercury is a heavy metal that's toxic to the human nervous system. Sadly, mercury has polluted our oceans and found its way into our seafood. Mercury exposure also comes from dental amalgam fillings (still!), as well as other areas of the environment. The detoxification of mercury and other heavy metals, such as lead, cadmium, and arsenic, deserves a full and separate discussion. For comprehensive and detailed information, check out the books by my friend and associate, Dr. Tom McGuire, which include *The Poison in Your Teeth: Mercury Amalgam (Silver) Fillings. . . Hazardous to Your*

Health!, *Healthy Teeth—Healthy Body*, and *Mercury Detoxification: The Natural Way to Remove Mercury from Your Body*.

The more general detoxification programs found in this book will support the elimination of mercury, lead, and other metal toxins. Natural elimination occurs when molecules stored in our tissues are determined to be toxic—our bodies continuously evaluate and expel such substances, and detoxing supports this process. Natural products like cilantro, garlic, and alginates (found in seaweeds) are helpful, and the medications dimercaptosuccinic acid (DMSA) and 2, 3-dimercapto-1-propanesulfonic acid (DMPS) are available by prescription (see the essay by Dr. McGuire on page 125). A product that I recommend and that has been shown to bind and remove heavy metals from the body is ZNatural, a naturally derived chelating water-soluble liquid compound from LifeHealth Sciences. ZNatural is approved by the FDA for daily use by consumers of all ages. You can learn more about ZNatural at the company's website, www.znatural.com.

EMOTIONAL CHALLENGES

Detoxification (and toxicity) occurs at every level of our being—physical, mental, emotional, and spiritual. As you progress through a detox program, your attitudes and feelings about your relationships at home, at work, and with the world at large may begin to shift. Now that you're *eating* differently, you may start *thinking* differently. And now that you're *behaving* differently (you're no longer smoking or drinking or overstimulating yourself with sugar and caffeine) you may find yourself *reacting* differently.

Be aware that this is a *perfectly normal* part of a healthy detoxification process!

Be aware, too, that those around you who aren't involved in the detox process may have strong feelings and opinions about what you're doing. How do you think your drinking buddies will feel when you're not drinking with them? Or the colleagues you used to take smoking or coffee breaks with? How will your attitudes toward them change? How about at home? Is it possible your spouse or partner might resent having to shop for and prepare meals differently? Although the detox process requires focusing on yourself, do try to be sensitive to and considerate of those around you. There will be emotional challenges along the way—and there may even be some casualties. Be prepared to make some difficult choices: you may need to let go of certain people, abandon particular environments, or stop engaging in certain activities that are no longer healthy for you.

The ultimate goal of my detoxification program is to give you the tools you need so that you do not revert to old destructive habits. The detox process is designed to help you reinvent your life in more healthful ways. To stay aligned with your new goals, it may be necessary to ask for support from family, friends, and colleagues. And it's up to you to be prepared

Mercury Concerns by Tom McGuire, DDS

Mercury is the most poisonous, naturally occurring, nonradioactive substance on the planet. One of the toxic heavy metals that includes lead, arsenic, and cadmium, it is commonly found in the environment. But according to the World Health Organization (WHO), the greatest exposure from mercury comes from dental amalgam fillings, contaminated fish and seafood, then other food sources, and air and water—in that order.

Mercury is classified as a neurotoxin, and chronic mercury poisoning (CMP) exhibits a great many symptoms related to the brain and central nervous system, including anxiety, depression, mood swings, and anger—just to name a few. CMP can have a devastating effect on the immune system and can directly, or indirectly, contribute to or make worse just about any health issue.

The harmful effects of mercury on the body make it very important to consider eliminating the main sources of mercury exposure, amalgam (silver) fillings and mercury-contaminated fish. Many suffering from CMP should consider participating in a mercury detoxification program designed to naturally and safely support the body's effort to remove accumulated mercury.

For information about mercury amalgam fillings, including their safe removal, and mercury detoxification I encourage you to check out the books that Dr. Haas has mentioned. I also have an extensive and informative website on these topics and from it you can access my books and the largest and most comprehensive Directory of Mercury-Safe Dentists (www.mercurysafedentists.com).

The more general detoxification programs discussed in Dr. Haas's *The Detox Diet* will also help support the elimination of mercury, other metals, and toxins. The body's detox (elimination) system is much more effective if we avoid the intake of all toxic substances (including mercury). The body has a full-time job dealing with what is already there and doesn't need an extra toxic burden.

In addition, because mercury is difficult to remove, it is critically important to support the body's natural elimination process. My detoxification program details the essential supplements necessary to help the body remove mercury, including natural products like cilantro and alginates (from seaweeds). Pharmaceutical mercury chelators that can bind with and remove mercury (and other heavy metals) include DMSA (meso-2, 3-dimercaptosuccinic acid) and DMPS (2,3-dimercapto-1-propane sulfonic acid) can also be effective in some situations (they require a medical prescription). Consult with your naturally oriented practitioner and mercury-safe dentist about mercury evaluation and detoxification.

for some resistance—and to be your own best advocate. With detoxification, it's not uncommon for participants to reevaluate and seek radical changes, not only in their diet but also in all aspects of their lives, including work and career choices, living situations, and interpersonal relationships. While this response is normal and very common, take it easy! It's much harder to undo a decision made in haste than it is to make a thoughtful, well-considered choice.

SPECIAL CIRCUMSTANCES

Detox and Travel

Detoxing is easier to do at home than while traveling for obvious reasons. But, it is possible to be away from home and on the move and still follow the basic guidelines. It's harder to steer clear of sugar, caffeine, dairy, and wheat if you're eating in fast food restaurants, so, if you can afford it, try to be choosy about where you dine. Upgrading your restaurant options usually means fewer unknowns in the nutrition equation, especially in terms of hygiene and food quality, and thus helps avoid food-borne illness. Focus on veggies, always!

Also, consider taking healthy snacks on the road, such as fresh fruit, nuts, seeds, trail mix, or nutrition bars. In short, whenever possible, plan ahead and be prepared.

Detoxing and Dining Out

Although dining out in a restaurant is often a challenge when it comes to avoiding sugar, salt, fats, wheat, cow's milk,

and so on, it can be done. Ask for what you want and let the waitperson know you have allergies to certain items. You can always order a salad with dressing on the side, rice with steamed or roasted vegetables, or fish or poultry with vegetables. Be sure to ask that any sauces or condiments be served on the side so you can control the amount you want, or decide to do without.

In my book, *Staying Healthy with Nutrition*, and on my website haashealthonline .com, there are suggested selections from a wide variety of restaurants.

LIVER DETOX

The liver is our detox organ; it is continuously detoxifying and eliminating metabolized toxins ingested with our food. The liver also produces thousands of substances our body uses. This extraordinary organ has a lot of responsibility and doesn't appreciate being overtaxed by its owner. Irresponsible food and substance choices make the liver's job more difficult. It's like asking an extremely busy person to do your job, too; she might do it, but she won't thank you for it.

Alcohol and petroleum by-products (contained in many cosmetics and perfumes) stress the liver and compromise many of its functions. Remove these substances from your body and you remove the stress on your liver. There are many products currently available that claim to support or heal the liver. But I've found that a good detox program is more effective. Herbs, such as dandelion root and leaf, burdock root, and milk thistle are safe and natural traditional liver remedies.

GALLBLADDER FLUSHES

There is a commonly misunderstood naturopathic practice that purports to dump many hundreds or even thousands of gallstones from the gallbladder. It prescribes a tonic of lemon juice and olive oil taken in the morning, followed by a period of time spent reclining on one's side and massaging the belly. The finale is the eventual passing of many white or green stonelike pebbles in our stool. And, wow, look at all those gallstones! The problem is they are not "stones" at all, but simply coagulated bits of oil and cholesterol and other flotsam or digestive tract material.

There are gallbladder and liver flushes available that may have some helpful organ-cleansing aspects; however, they do not clear stones. That said, olive oil supports a healthy liver, lemon is a natural cleanser, and both stimulate the release of bile from the gallbladder. While this natural "flush" doesn't actually clear gallstones either, it usually helps people feel better.

MIND POWER

To me, illness is the manifestation of a conflict in the mind and/or body; it represents the mind and body's call for some much-needed downtime. Resolving the

conflict through recovery and healing is up to us. Disease and/or healing occur at all levels of our being and are certainly influenced by how we think and live our lives. Further, scientific research shows that a positive optimistic attitude inspires healthier lifestyle choices and improved well-being. But without addressing attitudes and emotional challenges, it's difficult to make lifestyle changes. Having the strength to face these challenges comes from the inner wisdom to change how we view life and make the right choices, and the self-discipline to get great results.

In the beginning days of mind-body medicine, called psychoneuroimmunology or PNI, scientists started to investigate the role our mind plays in our health and our choices. In fact, a whole new field of positive psychology grew out of this. What has been shown is that what we think affects our emotional state, our choices, and our ability to change. The most exciting outcome is that we are able to change our negative attitudes to more positive ones through meditation, being in nature, music, laughter, and friendships. Our mind has power and although it takes effort to shift our thoughts, it's doable and worthwhile since they influence every part of our healthy living.

For a deeper exploration of my philosophies and approaches, review *Staying Healthy with the Seasons*, and my websites, haashealthonline.com and pmcmarin.com.

Part Two

BREAKING THE SNACC HABITS

Sugar, Nicotine, Alcohol, Caffeine, and Chemicals—or as I like to call them: **SNACCs**. They affect our energy, our moods, even our personalities through their stimulating or sedative effects. For those who have come to rely on any of these substances—part 2 is for you. My goal for you is to develop a healthy relationship with one or some or all of these common substances and/or the products that contain them.

Do you need two or three or more cups of coffee to get through your day? Do you routinely turn to sweet foods as a mood elevator? Do you use alcohol as a social lubricant or coping aid? Did you start smoking long before you understood the physiological addiction and consequences, and now cannot quit? Do you immediately reach into the medicine cabinet whenever you don't feel well? If you answered yes to any of these questions, this section will give you a better understanding of SNACCs, what they do, what they don't do, and how to extract them, so to speak, from your life.

Toxicity also comes from the environment and from personal relationships. Obviously, our environment is where we are exposed to many of the toxins from which we must detoxify. We have chemicals and metals that come into our body from the air, food, and water that we are exposed to or take in. In some ways, the beginning of the detox process has to do with lessening these exposures through chemical avoidance where possible—by drinking healthy water, eating noncontaminated and, as often as possible, organic foods, and making cleaner choices in the products we use on our skin and in our homes, because this is where many chemicals get into our bodies. Thus, dealing with our environment and the many exposures we have is part of everyone's life, both during each day and over the course of our many decades. To me, the biggest concern of modern living and for our long-term health is the buildup over time of environmental chemicals in our bodies.

Many people have toxic or problematic relationships. Assessing the health of our interactions with our spouses, sweethearts, kids, coworkers, and friends—and looking at what is disturbing or what can be corrected—is an important part of life and can be an integral part of detoxification and healing. Ideally, we never stop learning and growing as people.

During my groups' and many people's detox process, participants tune into and want to work on what feels out of balance in their most intimate relationships, helping better communication evolve in a healthy way. Of course, this is the topic of an entire book; here, I would simply point out that this healing of relationships can be a naturally occurring process that is part of the detox programs described in this book. During these programs, feelings and awareness may arise and need to be dealt with in each individual's relationship. Thus, I encourage spouses and families to do some of these programs together, which often brings them closer to each other and provides much-needed support.

CHAPTER TEN
Sugar Detoxification

FOR MOST OF US, sweetness symbolizes love and nurturance because our first food as infants is lactose, or milk sugar. Overconsumption and daily use of sugar is the first compulsive habit for most everyone with addictions later in life. Simple sugar, or glucose, is what our body, cells, and brain use as fuel for energy. Some glucose is stored in our liver and muscle tissues as glycogen for future use; excess sugar is stored as fat for use during periods of low-calorie intake or starvation.

Problems with sweets come from the frequency with which we eat them and the quantity of sugar we consume. The type of sugar we eat is also a contributing factor. Refined sugar or sucrose (a disaccharide made up of two simple sugars—glucose and fructose) is usually extracted from sugarcane or sugar beets, initially whole foods. However, most all of the nutrients are removed and retained only in the discarded extract called molasses. When the manufacturing process is complete, the result is pure sugar, a refined crystal that contains four calories per gram and essentially no nutrients.

Sugar and sweeteners have so pervaded our food-manufacturing and restaurant industries that it is almost impossible to find prepackaged products that are unsweetened. Most frequently used are refined, high-calorie, non-nutrient sucrose and corn syrup derivatives, mainly as high-fructose corn syrup. Consequently, the only way to avoid sweeteners is to avoid packaged products and recipes with sugar whenever possible. Fruits contain natural fructose, in balance with other nutrients; honey and maple syrup are more highly concentrated natural sugars and are appropriate for most of us in moderation because they are all sources of sugar (carbohydrate) calories.

Traditional Chinese medicine views the desire for sugar, or the sweet flavor, as a craving for the mother (yin) energy, a craving that represents a need for comfort or security. A desire for spicy or salty flavored foods might represent looking for the father (yang) energy, or power and direction. In Western cultures, we have turned sugar into a reward system (a tangible symbol of nurturing) to the degree that many of us have been conditioned to need some sweet treat to feel complete or satisfied. We continue these patterns with our children, unconsciously showing our affection for them by giving them sugary foods. Holidays and special occasions are centered around sugar—birthday cakes and ice cream, Halloween candy, chocolate Easter eggs, Thanksgiving pie, Christmas cookies, Valentine's Day chocolates—the list is endless. We even reward our children for good behavior by giving them treats. Sweet talk is embedded in our language—sweetie, sweetie pie, sweetheart, honey, honey pie, sugar, sugar baby, candy, sweet cakes, baby cakes, honey bun, sugar plum, and so on. The message is loud and clear: **sweetness = love.**

POTENTIAL PROBLEMS ASSOCIATED WITH SUGAR INTAKE

- Tooth decay

- Obesity and increased risk of diabetes, cancer, and other diseases

- Nutritional deficiency, including anemia, protein, and mineral deficiencies

- Hypoglycemia and carbohydrate imbalance

- Chronic dyspepsia and digestive problems

- Immune dysfunction and problems such as recurrent infections

- Menstrual irregularities and premenstrual symptoms (PMS)

- Yeast overgrowth and its many subsequent problems, including craving sweets and carbohydrates

- Hyperactivity and difficulty concentrating

- Alcoholism and its potential link to hypoglycemia and abnormal carbohydrate metabolism

- Mood swings, anxiety, and depression

- Heart disease

There is much evidence that eating too many sweets eventually causes disease. However, it is also the corresponding lack of physical activity that complicates the problem, eventually affecting weight and health. If any of these problems are part of your personal or family history, it is important to seriously consider a dietary change for your health's sake.

SUGAR AND HEALTH

Many nutritional authorities feel that the high use of sugar in our diet is a significant underlying cause of obesity and many diseases. Too much sweetener in any form can have a negative effect on our health; this includes not only refined sugar but also corn syrup, honey, fruit juices, and treats such as sodas, cakes, and candies. Because sugary foods briefly satisfy our hunger, they often replace more nutritious foods and weaken our bodies' health and disease resistance.

Sugar can also compromise the body's ability to fight illness and may alter immune defenses. Recent studies indicate that people who have high blood sugar levels are five times more likely to experience post-surgical infections than people with blood sugar levels less than 140 mg/dl.[1] In a number of other studies, researchers found a positive association between high blood sugar levels and an increased incidence of cancer. However, many researchers conclude it is the insulin that increases with sugar consumption that is the likely culprit, not the sugar.[2] A Korean study found a greater incidence of cancer among people who were diabetic.[3]

A connection between high sugar intake and coronary artery disease has been speculated since the 1960s. Research since then strongly suggests that a high carbohydrate diet puts women at greater risk than men for the development of cardiovascular disease.[4] And for women who take birth control pills or hormones, the risk may be higher.

Increased sugar consumption can lead to impaired glucose tolerance, one of the strongest predictors of type 2 (previously known as adult-onset or non-insulin-dependent) diabetes. With type 1 or insulin-dependent diabetes, positive actions to manage sugar and starch intake can help protect against associated secondary problems, such as neuropathy and blindness. People with diabetes of any sort need to take special measures to keep their carbohydrate intake low.

Many people are sensitive to dietary sugars and experience digestive upset and chronic indigestion from excessive intake of sweets. *Candida albicans* and other microorganisms love sweet, simple, sugary foods. A sweet diet encourages greater infestation of bacteria, yeasts, and parasites, and will support their growth orally and in the rest of the digestive tract.[5] Microbe infestation can also weaken our immunity. In addition, the presence of candida and other unfriendly organisms in our gut or other organ systems increases our craving for sweets, creating and perpetuating a negative cycle.

Frequent cravings for sweets can also be related to hypoglycemia (low blood sugar). Chronic low blood sugar can be the result of poor adrenal and pancreatic function. However, we all get low blood sugar from time to time, when we skip a meal or work extra hard. If our blood sugar is low, a candy bar, a piece of cake, a cup of sweetened coffee, or an alcoholic beverage furnishes a quick pick-me-up, reducing the symptoms of shakiness, fatigue, or anxiety. However, this relief is only short term. Sugar is absorbed so rapidly into the blood that the pancreas overreacts to balance the glucose level. This can cause a rapid drop in blood sugar, which may result in mood swings with depression or anger. Orthomolecular Medicine has suggested that some alcoholism may result from such hypoglycemic (low blood sugar) mood swings. In such cases, continuing to drink alcohol keeps the blood sugar up and the anxiety level down, but with negative long-term effects.

Sugar cravings are commonly experienced by women premenstrually, and chocolate is a common first choice to appease that craving. In Traditional Chinese medicine, the regular use or overuse of sugar is thought to lead to menstrual irregularities and premenstrual problems, such as pain, swelling, and irritability.

Sugar excess may also cause our bodies to age more rapidly. In 1993, geriatric researchers found high-calorie intake (from all food) to be a significant dietary factor responsible for aging. Empty calories from sweeteners and sweet foods may give us quick energy, but they also increase our energy utilization that stresses and ages our bodies more rapidly.

Our teeth are also subject to the destructive effects of sugar. When refined sugar was introduced into the diets of native peoples, such as the Inuit of North

---

SUGAR CULPRITS

Food groups that contribute the largest portions of added sugars to the American diet, as a percentage of total added sugars consumed. These are defined as sugars and syrups added to foods during processing or preparation, or at the table.

Regular soft drinks	33.0%
Sugars and candy	16.1%
Cakes, cookies, pies	12.9%
Fruit drinks (-ades and punch)	9.7%
Dairy desserts and milk products (ice cream, sweetened yogurt, sweetened milk)	8.6%
Other grains (cinnamon toast, honey-nut waffles)	5.8%

Source: American Heart Association

America, New Zealand's Maoris, and Australia's aborigines, the number of dental cavities increased dramatically; whereas in Europe and Japan, when sugar was rationed during World War II, the rate of cavities fell significantly. Research consistently shows that sugar and sticky starches destroy dental enamel and cause plaque and decay. Sweetened beverages are also linked to increased cavities. A major U.S. survey found that the use of soft drinks or sweet juices three or more times per day between meals doubled the chances of developing cavities.

SUGAR AND ITS EFFECTS ON CHILDREN

Lifetime dietary habits are formed in infancy, so limiting the intake of sweets at this developmental stage is of major importance. Blood sugar levels during infancy are less stable than later in childhood; thus babies are more susceptible to foods that rapidly raise and lower blood sugar. In fact, infant failure-to-thrive syndrome has been correlated with impaired carbohydrate metabolism, and specifically sucrose malabsorption. Some babies and young children develop chronic colic, cramping,

Sugar Alternatives

The sweetener called Just Like Sugar is a good sugar alternative because it does not have a laxative effect, contains no calories, and provides 200 mg of fiber per teaspoon. The fiber in Just Like Sugar is inulin from chicory root, which is a prebiotic fiber that actually supports the growth of the good bacteria (microflora or probiotic) in the intestines, thereby improving digestion. Chicory inulin is a nondigestible oligosaccharide, which means it passes through the digestive system without being absorbed, so it doesn't provide calories. This is beneficial because other sweeteners such as cane sugar and beet sugar are laden with calories, with the potential for becoming body fat when taken in excess. Also those sugars cause inflammation, which is damaging to blood vessels. So this sweetener wins in two ways, not only because it does no harm but also because it improves digestion. Oh, and it really does taste just like sugar.

Natural sweeteners are those extracted from natural foods like honey, maple syrup, agave nectar, malt, and rice syrup. They are primarily whole foods. Beets, sugarcane, and corn are derived used to make "sugar" and corn syrup, yet this is more processed, "refined," and only a portion of the food, with more sugar calories and not many nutrients.

and diarrhea from eating sugar, and this has been reported in the medical literature for more than twenty years.

Learning problems, exaggerated hyperactivity, and moodiness in children have all been linked to a high-sugar diet. Psychologists have observed decreased performance and increased inappropriate behavior following sugar intake. Many school teachers and mothers believe in this sugar-behavior relationship. This whole issue remains controversial. For certain children with ADHD (Attention Deficit Hyperactivity Disorder), these effects can be more extreme. Not surprisingly, researchers found that decreasing sugar decreased socially inappropriate behavior. Yet in a Korean study of fifth-grade children, they found no significant association between total simple sugar intake from snacks and ADHD development.[6]

The long-term effects of a sweet diet may actually be more severe than the immediate concerns. The habits we establish when we are young set the stage for lifetime patterns. A diet of empty calories may be a factor in frequent infections and failure to thrive. Extensive childhood dental cavities may result in teeth damaged beyond repair as an adult. Hypoglycemia in youth may result in recurring depression or alcoholism later in life. Chronic candida (yeast) infections, resulting from the frequent intake of sweets and the use of antibiotics, may set the stage for a lifetime of digestive and energy problems. In recent decades, childhood obesity has gotten out of hand and has tripled in the past twenty to thirty years. Overweight children may become overweight adults, with the attendant increased risks for diabetes, cancer, and heart disease.

DECREASING THE SUGAR IN OUR DIET

Our intake of sweets is increasing, especially because of the addition of hidden sweeteners in our foods. A quick look at the yearly statistics gives the impression that we are eating fewer sweets, because our annual per capita consumption of beet and cane sugar has dropped from about 72 pounds in 1970 to 47 pounds in 2010.[7] Sounds good. However, within the same time frame, our yearly intake of high-fructose corn syrup has gone from less than 0.5 pound to 35 pounds per person. Add another 12 pounds for other natural sweeteners. Our total intake of sweeteners is now almost 100 pounds a year per person—and that's not including artificial sweeteners.

Reducing sweeteners in our diet is a very real, positive step each of us can take. It requires an effort, but reducing our dietary load of sugar and sweeteners is of key importance for our health and our children's health. The most popular zero-calorie artificial sweetener, aspartame (NutraSweet and Equal), is not a worthy replacement. This substance can be a neurological irritant and affect a user's mood and energy. It should not be used by people who have phenylketonuria or in large

AVOID SUGAR FOODS AND SNACKS

White sugar	Candy	Cake
Soda pop	Artificial juices	Sweetened drinks
Pies	Puddings	Cookies
Ice cream	Doughnuts	Breakfast cereals
Gelatin	Corn syrup	Liqueurs
Jams and jellies	Chewing gum	Mixed drinks

AVOID HIDDEN SUGAR IN FOODS

Baking mixes	Breads	Crackers
Ketchup	Relish	Tartar sauce
Salad dressings	Cheese dips	Soups
Pickles	Peanut butter	Frankfurters
Luncheon meats	Prepared seafood	Sausage
Canned fruits	Frozen vegetables	Sweetened yogurt

CALORIC SUGAR SUBSTANCES ADDED TO FOODS

Sucrose	Fructose	Dextrose
Glucose	Honey	Malt syrup
Maple sugar/syrup	Corn syrup	Corn sweetener
High-fructose corn syrup	Lactose	Maltose
Brown sugar	Molasses	Agave nectar

quantities by anyone. It also interacts with other foods and changes their taste. Although in some studies, aspartame is reported to have limited toxicity, I have seen many people who do not tolerate this nonsugar sweetener in similar ways that people do not tolerate MSG (monosodium glutamate, the flavor enhancer used commonly in Chinese cooking), with agitation and headaches.[8]

Sorbitol, mannitol, erythitol, and xylitol are generally better tolerated and safer. However, these alcohol-type sweeteners are not well absorbed by the intestines, so in excess they may cause gas and loose stools. Stevia is a natural alternative sweetener that is now widely available. It is a commercial preparation from an herb that many diabetics can use without risk of raising blood sugar levels. However, some studies suggest it can also lower blood sugar levels and make glucose control difficult in diabetics.[9] Side effects can include bloating, nausea, and dizziness. People with allergies to ragweed and related plants could have allergic reactions to stevia.[10]

THE GLYCEMIC INDEX

Sometimes referred to as the glycemic load, the glycemic index is a relatively new concept that relates to how quickly any sugars in foods are absorbed into the bloodstream from the digestive tract. Basically, all simple sugars absorb quickly by themselves, with alcohol (a type of sugar) being absorbed quite rapidly. High-glycemic foods are absorbed quickly, and lower-glycemic foods, like oatmeal, are absorbed less quickly. Review the list on the next page, and you may be a bit surprised at what foods are high or low on the glycemic chart. If you eat foods lower on the glycemic index, your blood sugar will

CASE STUDY: JEFF, AGE 52

On our way to be Earth Guardian assistants for the last and most easterly stand of redwoods in Redwood Valley, California, we were joined by a local realtor and her brother. During our journey, the tragic tale of her brother Jeff and his family was shared with us.

Two months prior, Jeff's wife of many years and the mother of his child had committed suicide. Jeff moved in with his sister and spent his days lying on the couch with zero motivation. Of course, he had suffered a devastating loss.

His sister shared her observations. She saw her brother consuming more than a six-pack of diet soda daily, including having a can at his bedside in a cooler at all times, which he drank throughout the night. She said, "Jeff, it's pretty clear you're not doing very well. Do you ever drink water or juice or anything else?" Jeff replied, "Not really."

Now here's the story that he relayed. Two years prior, he and his wife had realized that they had gained a little too much weight. They began a diet and included diet sodas to replace their use of sugar. They also added packets of the sweetener aspartame to other foods and beverages. Over the next few months, their moods began to shift and they became more and more depressed. They consulted a doctor who prescribed antidepressants for both of them. Without significant results, two other medicines were added over the next few months. None of their physicians interviewed them about their lifestyle habits.

As their moods and emotions became worse, one day Jeff came home and found a note next to the body of his wife who had shot and killed herself. "I can't go on, please care for our daughter." With this crisis, the daughter stayed with other relatives, and Jeff went to stay with his sister.

In response to the question about his diet soda use, they agreed to try an experiment. He shifted to drinking water and juice for several days. On the third day, he got off the couch and began washing and cleaning his car. Each day he began to feel better, and his mood became more positive. He was tapered off his medication and is now medicine- and diet soda–free and is actively participating in life. He believes, as I do, that he was having a reaction to the aspartame, which affected his mood and nervous system. This is not uncommon, although this case is, of course, extreme.

This experience has inspired me to write a new book about the health-care system and how doctors can be more attentive to finding the real causes of most health problems.

As practitioners, if we do not explore with our patients their lifestyle choices and what effect each activity has on their energy, moods, and relationships, we cannot begin to address these important issues. If we only treat end results with medicines, and not address the underlying causes, then we are not practicing to the best of our capabilities.

We can clearly do better, and that is what my books and life work are dedicated to—educating both patients and health-care practitioners to address and correct the true causes of illness.

And, by the way, the redwood forest was saved by a local angel investor.

GLYCEMIC INDEX OF CARBOHYDRATE FOODS

Note: Eating low on the index makes everything a little easier.

Any food below 55 on the glycemic index tends to conserve insulin and hormones. Overeating usually isn't a problem. It's the blast of insulin from foods high on the index that drives hunger cravings. With a diet of whole foods, appetite seems to drop quite naturally.

Grains, Breads, and Cereals

White bread	95
Instant rice	90
Rice cakes	80
Pretzels	80
Cornflakes	75
White flour	75
Graham crackers	75
Regular crackers	75
White bagel	75
Cheerios	75
Puffed wheat	75
White rice	70
Taco shells	70
Spaghetti	60
Pita bread	55
Wild rice/brown rice	55
Oatmeal	55
Popcorn	55
Nuts	15 to 30

Fruits

Watermelon	70
Pineapple	65
Raisins	65 to 95
Ripe bananas	60
Mango, kiwi, grapes	50
Pears	45
Peaches, plums	40
Apples, oranges	40
Dried apricots	30 to 70
Grapefruit	25
Cherries	25

Vegetables

Baked potato	95
Parsnips	95
Carrots	85
French fries	80
Corn (sweet)	75
Beets	70
Sweet potatoes	55
Yams	50
Green peas	45
Green beans	45
Pinto beans	40
Lima beans	40
Butter beans	30
Black beans	30
Kidney beans	30
Artichoke	25
Asparagus	20
Tomatoes	15
Green vegetables	15

Dairy Products

Ice cream, premium	60
Yogurt, with fruit	35
Milk, whole	30+
Milk, low-fat	30
Yogurt, plain, no sugar	15

Sweeteners

Maltose	105 to 150
Glucose	100
Honey	75
Refined sugar	75

Adapted from several sources, including *30-40-40: Fat-Burning Nutrition* by Joyce Daoust and *Sugar Busters* by Dr. Steward, et al.

SUGAR DETOXIFICATION NUTRIENT PROGRAM

	Adults	Children
Water	2 to 3 qt	1 to 2 qt
Fiber	20 to 40 g	10 to 20 g
Vitamin E	200 to 800 IU	50 to 100 IU
Thiamine (B$_1$)	25 to 100 mg	10 to 50 mg
Riboflavin (B$_2$)	25 to 100 mg	10 to 25 mg
Niacinamide (B$_3$)	50 to 100 mg	10 to 50 mg
Pantothenic acid (B$_5$)	250 to 1,000 mg	50 to 100 mg
Pyridoxine (B$_6$)	25 to 100 mg	10 to 25 mg
Cobalamin (B$_{12}$)	100 to 250 mcg	25 to 100 mcg
Folic acid	400 to 800 mcg	200 to 400 mcg
Vitamin C	2 to 10 g	500 to 1,000 mg
Bioflavonoids	250 to 500 mg	100 to 250 mg
Calcium	650 to 1,200 mg	350 to 600 mg
Chromium	400 to 1,000 mcg	100 to 250 mcg
Magnesium	400 to 800 mg	200 to 400 mg
Manganese	5 to 10 mg	3 to 5 mg
Selenium	200 to 300 mcg	50 to 100 mcg
Vanadium	200 to 400 mcg	50 to 100 mcg
Zinc	30 to 60 mg	15 to 30 mg
L-amino acids	1,000 to 1,500 mg	250 to 500 mg
L-glutamine	500 to 1,000 mg	250 to 500 mg
Essential fatty acids, such as flaxseed or fish oils	2 to 4 capsules	2 capsules
Adrenal glandular	100 to 200 mg	0

I believe sugar is the number one addiction on our planet. Take a break some time and see how you feel. You may feel more real.

be more stable. When your blood sugar level is stable, you will feel more energetic and likely experience less fatigue as well as less frequent mood shifts. Although we may strive to eat foods that are glycemically low, most of us end up eating some of the foods that are higher on the glycemic index now and then. Just be sure to eat them with high-fiber, slower absorbing starches or, more importantly, some protein and/or fat-containing food, such as a few almonds. For example, if you eat rice cakes, which are relatively high on the glycemic index, be sure to add nut butter (peanut butter, almond butter, cashew butter, and so forth), albacore tuna, or avocado slices, which are glycemically lower to help the rice cakes digest more slowly.

Low-carbohydrate diets are quite popular for weight loss these days, but there is a concern with excessive protein (and fats in some). Yet, there are healthy carbs (the complex starches and the high-fiber whole grains) and fattening ones (the sugars and refined flour products). I suggest a diet with a good balance of wholesome foods that include fruits and whole grains along with lots of vegetables, some nuts and seeds, and individually needed proteins.

SUGAR DETOX

Although sugar addiction is common, sugar withdrawal is usually physically mild, with periodic strong cravings. Emotional attachments and withdrawals may be more pronounced. For those who are sensitive to refined sugar or sweeteners, or who consume them in large amounts, genuine symptoms of abuse and withdrawal may occur. Some of these symptoms include fatigue, anxiety and irritability, depression and detachment, rapid heart rate and palpitations, and poor sleep. Most symptoms, if they do occur, last only a few days.

We can decide to cut down on or eliminate sugar quite easily by simply avoiding many of the sweet foods. There are plenty of nutritious nibbles to replace sugary snacks or treats—see page 138 for suggestions. We should clear our cupboards of unhealthy sweetened foods. Once sugar has been removed from the diet, it is still possible to use it once in a while, as it is not as readdicting as many stronger drugs. Most people who have kicked the sugar habit find that they no longer tolerate sugar very well.

A diet that is rich in whole grains and other complex carbohydrates, vegetables, and protein foods can also help stabilize blood sugar and minimize the desire for sugar. Many people who are protein deficient seem to crave sugars and carbohydrate foods. Conversely, eating a diet that focuses on protein and vegetables is a good way to minimize sugar cravings. If you don't tolerate sugars and sweet foods well, fruits should also be minimized and fruit juice avoided.

SUPPLEMENTS AND SUGAR

Nutrients that can help reduce sugar cravings and the symptoms of sugar withdrawal are the B vitamins, vitamin C, zinc, the trace mineral chromium, and the amino acid L-glutamine. Chromium is a cofactor in helping insulin work more efficiently in removing sugar from the blood and nourishing the cells. L-glutamine, which can be used directly as a fuel source in the body and brain, is also helpful in reducing sugar (and alcohol) cravings.

Children can also benefit from a nutritional supplement program that includes some of the above-mentioned nutrients, of course in lower amounts than for adults. Use of a good quality children's multiple vitamin-mineral, additional B vitamins to support the nervous system and general development, vitamin C at about 250 mg twice daily, and extra chromium (50 to 100 mcg one to two times daily) all help minimize sugar cravings and the transition from sugar and sweetened foods. The supplement plan applies to children ages six to eleven; amounts may vary depending

---

OVERCOMING A SWEET TOOTH

1. **Take sugar overconsumption seriously**—it can have insidious negative effects over time. This is particularly true for young people later in their lives.

2. **Eat a diet that includes vegetables,** whole grains (complex carbohydrates), and protein. Increasing protein levels in the diet, both animal and vegetable, helps reduce sugar cravings and use.

3. If you seriously overuse sugar, **omit it** (at least take a break to better understand your relationship to sugar) and consciously limit your intake of "hidden sweeteners" (particularly refined sugar [sucrose], corn syrup, and dextrose), and limit your use of honey and maple syrup. Eat some fruit, if you tolerate it, for natural sugar.

4. Support your body with **extra helpful nutrients**—these include the B vitamins, vitamin C, chromium, calcium, magnesium, and the amino acid L-glutamine.

5. **Drink 8 glasses of water** or herbal tea a day.

6. **Get sufficient fiber** to keep your body cleansed and light.

7. If you suspect that you are hypoglycemic or diabetic, **request the appropriate tests**—such as a fasting blood sugar or a 5- or 6-hour glucose tolerance test—from your health-care practitioner.

on the age and size of each child. These vitamins are water soluble and basically nontoxic. However, if your child has a special problem or is below the age of six, you should check with your pediatrician or health-care provider for specific recommendations.

The use of sugar in our culture resembles the use of a drug and can be treated as such. Make a clear plan for withdrawal while working on your emotions to eliminate the habit. Responses to flavors, certain food compulsions, and the feelings we get from them are usually conditioned. Self-reflection can be valuable. To change our habits, to stop and see things clearly, or to talk them through helps us transition from compulsion to the safe and balanced use of foods, sugar, and sweetened foods, as well as other substances we may use in our life.

Endnotes

1. Ashar Ata et al., "High Blood Sugar Levels Increase Infection Risk from General Surgery," *Archives of Surgery* 145, no. 9 (September 2010): 858–64.

2. P.J. Goodwin et al., "Fasting Insulin and Outcome in Early-Stage Breast Cancer: Results of a Prospective Cohort Study," *Journal of Clinical Oncology* 20 (2002): 42–51.

3. S.H. Jee et al., "Fasting Serum Glucose Level and Cancer Risk in Korean Men and Women," *Journal of the American Medical Association* 293, no. 2 (January 12, 2005): 194–202.

4. S. Sieri et al., "Dietary Glycemic Load and Index and Risk of Coronary Heart Disease in a Large Italian Cohort: the EPICOR Study. Results Risk Increased in Women Not Men," *Archives of Internal Medicine* 170, no. 7 (April 12, 2010): 640–7.

5. G. Pizzo, "Effect of Dietary Carbohydrates on the in Vitro Epithelial Adhesion of *Candida albicans*, *Candida tropicalis*, and *Candida krusei*," *New Microbiologica* 23, no. 1 (January 2000): 63–71.

6. Y. Kim and H. Chang, "Correlation Between Attention Deficit Hyperactivity Disorder and Sugar Consumption, Quality of Diet, and Dietary Behavior in School Children," *Nutrition Research and Practice* 5, no. 3 (June 2011): 236–45.

7. USDA May 2011 report, www.ers.usda.gov/briefing/sugar/data.htm

8. B.A. Magnuson et al., "Aspartame: A Safety Evaluation Based on Current Use Levels, Regulations, and Toxicological and Epidemiological Studies," *Critical Reviews in Toxicology* 37, no. 8 (2007): 629–727.

9. S. Gregersen et al., "Antihyperglycemic Effects of Stevioside in Type 2 Diabetic Subjects," *Metabolism* 53 (2004): 73–6.

10. www.webmd.com/vitamins-supplements/ingredientmono-682-STEVIA.aspx?activeIngredientId=682&activeIngredientName=STEVIA.

CHAPTER ELEVEN
Nicotine Detoxification

THE CIGARETTE IS ONE OF THE world's most profitable globally distributed substances. Why? Because nicotine is more addictive than either alcohol or cocaine; thus people cannot stop and must keep buying cigarettes, even when they have little money for food and other necessities. However, in recent years the U.S. courts and ordinary citizens have made the cigarette companies pay big money back to the smokers who have been injured from smoking addiction. Nicotine pushers didn't tell the public that smoking was so addictive. They still downplay this fact and appear to have little concern about getting new customers hooked on their product (except to get new customers hooked on their product). While widespread education and growing awareness about the dangers of tobacco has contributed to fewer people starting across all age groups, tobacco use remains the leading preventable cause of death.[1] Cigarette use probably creates the most difficult addiction to deal with.

The statistics are shocking: Worldwide, 5 to 6 million people per year die of tobacco-related diseases.[2] In the United States alone, cigarette smoking accounts for more than a half million deaths each year. Plus there are another 8 million people who live with serious disease caused by cigarette smoking. Most data do not include tobacco use in other forms such as cigars, pipes, smokeless tobacco, and chewing.[3] Among teens, marijuana use continues to rise while alcohol and tobacco abuse lessens. And tobacco use is declining in the United States, but increasing in low-income countries.

In the United States, cigarette smoking is responsible for more 30 percent of cancer deaths and 30 percent of heart disease deaths.[4] See the chart

443,000 ANNUAL U.S. DEATHS ATTRIBUTABLE TO CIGARETTE SMOKING*

Lung cancer	128,000
Ischemic heart disease	126,000
Chronic obstructive pulmonary disease (COPD)	92,000
Other diagnoses	44,000
Other cancers	35,300
Stroke	19,500

* Annual average number of deaths, 2000–2004. Source: *Morbidity and Mortality Weekly Report* 57, no. 45 (2008): 1226–1228.

above for the statistics. We here in the States have fewer than 10 percent of the world's deaths associated with nicotine addiction, which means smoking health issues and death from nicotine are a worldwide concern, and cost countries billions. Europe and parts of Asia have even higher rates of smoking than we do, stressing health-care systems everywhere. When I was in Ghana, Africa, recently, I saw no local people smoking, just travelers from the United States and Europe.

Cigarette smoking also increases the incidence of atherosclerosis, strokes, and peripheral vascular disease. Diseases of the respiratory tract, colds, flu, acute bronchitis, pneumonia, chronic obstructive pulmonary diseases (COPD) such as emphysema and chronic bronchitis, and of course, lung cancer—are all much more common in smokers. Infections and allergies are also prevalent in smokers, as is rapid aging of the body, especially facial

skin, which results from the poor oxygenation of tissues and other associated chemical effects.

Smoking clearly decreases life expectancy for all age groups. One-pack-a-day smokers double their chance of death between ages fifty and sixty, while two-packers triple theirs. Both health and life insurance rates are more for smokers than nonsmokers. (Smokers may pay twice that of nonsmokers.) Smoking also affects the life expectancy of family nonsmokers.[5] An estimated 88 million nonsmoking Americans, including children aged three to eleven years, are exposed to secondhand smoke.[6] Fortunately, the trends for smoking are decreasing each year across all age groups.[7] Still, of all the commonly used drugs, nicotine has the least benefits and the greatest consequences.

The economic burden of tobacco use in the United States is more than $96 billion a year in medical costs and another

$97 billion a year from lost productivity.[8] The 2009/2010 report from the National Cancer Institute stated that in 2008 the average age for first use among those aged twelve to seventeen years was fifteen years. Among those aged eighteen to twenty-five, the average age at first use was almost nineteen.[9] Most smokers try their first cigarette before they are eighteen and become addicted as adolescents. Recent estimates suggest that about 21 percent of the over-eighteen population in the United States smokes.[10] More men smoke (23.5 percent) than women (17.9 percent). Percentages of adult smokers are much higher in most European countries and parts of Asia. Billions of dollars are spent to treat the problems that afflict smokers, and many more billions are lost due to decreased work and productivity. Many countries, including the United States, have invested in substantial and effective programs to help people stop smoking and to never start.

Childhood addiction to cigarettes is the saddest part of the nicotine story. We must continue to insist on more stringent laws to better regulate sales and advertising, along with better education to help curtail this problem. One of the salient points arising from basic research is this: Tobacco smoking causes an important gene mutation to the p53 or tumor suppressor gene system, making the smoker much more vulnerable to cancer. For people who started smoking as adults and stop, this mutation is reversible, lowering their risk for cancer. However, for people who started

smoking as adolescents, the gene damage is permanent.[11]

Since most nicotine is ingested by smoking cigarettes, that is the focus of this chapter. Cigar and pipe smoking, chewing tobacco, and snuff also pose health risks, but far fewer than with cigarettes. Tobacco comes from a large-leafed nightshade, or *Solanaceae*, plant. It is one of only a few plants that contain the psychoactive alkaloid nicotine. Tobacco and eating plants from the nightshade family (white potatoes, tomatoes, and peppers) causes joint pain in some people, which correlates with the theory that arthritis is in part due to nightshade sensitivity.

The highly addictive nature of nicotine is revealed by the fact that many strong-minded and strong-willed people cannot stop smoking, even if they are otherwise health conscious. Over 80 percent of smokers say that they want to stop. In my years working in hospitals, I saw lung cancer and emphysema patients smoking between ventilator treatments and patients with tubes in their necks from tracheostomies putting cigarettes into the tubes to inhale.

The initial irritating effects of nicotine easily progress to chronic irritations, yet these are outweighed by the physiological and psychological dependence. People addicted to heroin and other powerful drugs have commonly cited nicotine as the hardest drug to kick. The American Psychiatric Association has described smoking as an organic mental disorder. Their statistics suggest that around 50 percent of people cannot stop smoking when they try to and that of the people who do stop, about 75 percent of them begin again within one year.

NICOTINE EFFECTS AND BENEFITS (YES, THERE ARE A FEW)

Many people find smoking to be relaxing, but this may be related to the way it calms hyperactive withdrawal symptoms. People do experience increased mental stimulation and improved hand-eye coordination as a result of nicotine's vascular-neurological stimulation, but the effects do not last. The "up" feeling that smoking produces is more likely correlated with increased blood pressure and heart rate, as well as the production of fatty acids, steroids, hormones, and neurotransmitters (and easing from withdrawal). Nicotine mimics acetylcholine, which improves alertness, memory, and learning capacity. Stimulation of norepinephrine and endorphins by nicotine may help balance moods and increase energy. The liver's increased glycogen release gives a satisfying lift to the blood sugar.

Dr. Tom Ferguson's book *The Smoker's Book of Health* cites how hundreds of smokers said they felt better able to deal with stress and to relax with nicotine.[12] Smoking helped control their moods, improved concentration and energy levels (especially with fatigue), and reduced withdrawal symptoms. Social comfort, work breaks, reduced pain and anxiety,

increased pleasure, and less boredom were also noted.

Smoking also reduces one's appetite and taste for food, a benefit for the weight conscious. In fact, the average smoker weighs 6 to 8 pounds less than the nonsmoker. And when he or she quits smoking, the average smoker gains about 15 pounds.[13] In the book *Life Extension* (currently out of print), Sandy Shaw and Durk Pearson note that nicotine seems to reduce distraction by outside stimuli in people working in highly stimulating environments—that is, it desensitizes people.

Nicotine is a mild central nervous system stimulant and a strong cardiovascular system stimulant. It constricts blood vessels, increasing blood pressure and stimulating the heart, and raises blood fat levels. In its liquid form, nicotine is a powerful poison—the injection of even one drop would be deadly. Interestingly, it is the nicotine, not the smoke, that causes people to continue smoking cigarettes, yet it is the smoking itself that causes so many of the health problems. The average cigarette contains about 1 mg of absorbable nicotine, though manufacturers keep on increasing the amount; a dose of 40 to 60 mg could be lethal to humans.[14]

Although people love their cigarettes and smoking breaks and actually feel "up" and stimulated, we all know now that the hazards and damage are quite costly and far outweigh any possible benefits.

WHAT ARE THE RISKS OF SMOKING?

Cigarette smoke is a combination of lethal gases (carbon monoxide, hydrogen cyanide, and nitrogen and sulfur oxides) and tars (which contain an estimated four thousand chemicals). Some of these chemical agents are introduced by the actual manufacturing processes. Tobacco has been smoked for centuries, and until recently it has been naturally grown and dried. It appears that in the last century, as chemicals have been added, the negative effects of smoking have skyrocketed. Research suggests that natural tobacco poses much less cancer and cardiovascular disease risk than processed tobacco does.

Dangers in modern tobacco products include pesticides used during cultivation and chemicals added to the tobacco to make it burn better or taste different. Chemicals added to the leaves and papers to enhance burning are a major cause of fire death in this country, because those cigarettes continue to burn after they have been set down or dropped when the person has fallen asleep while smoking. Forced burning also makes people smoke more of each cigarette in order to keep up with it. Sugar curing and rapid flue drying are also associated with increased toxicity. Kerosene heat drying contaminates the tobacco with yet another toxic hydrocarbon. If a cigarette does not go out when left alone, it has been chemically treated. Using a natural tobacco (organic, such as American Spirit) may reduce smoking

risks, although it doesn't eliminate the dangers of smoking.

Other toxic contaminants in cigarettes include cadmium (which affects the kidneys, arteries, and blood pressure), lead, arsenic, cyanide, and nickel. Dioxin, one of the most toxic pesticide chemicals known has been found in cigarettes, as has acetonitrile, another pesticide.[15] The nitrogen gases from cigarettes generate carcinogenic nitrosamines in body tissues. The tars in smoke contain polynuclear aromatic hydrocarbons (PAH), carcinogenic materials that bind with cellular DNA to cause damage. Antioxidant therapy, particularly with vitamin C, helps protect against both PAH and nitrosamines. Extra vitamin C blocks the irritating effects of smoke and replaces what is lost due to reduced absorption (blood levels of ascorbic acid average about 30 to 40 percent lower in smokers than in nonsmokers).

Radioactive materials are also found in cigarette smoke, lead and polonium being the most common.[16] For longtime smokers, cigarettes can be the greatest source of accumulated radiation, which is a strong aging factor. Smoking one pack of cigarettes per day for a year exposes the smoker to 0.36 millisieverts, equivalent to the radiation from one mammogram or seventy-two dental X-rays.[17] Acetaldehyde, a chemical released during smoking, also causes aging (especially of the skin) because it is an irritant.

There are different levels of nicotine addiction. Least addicted are those who smoke socially—only at parties with

PROBLEMS ASSOCIATED WITH SMOKING

Cough
Hoarseness
Headaches
Anxiety
Fatigue
Leg pains
Cold hands and feet
Memory loss
Senility
Alzheimer's disease
Rapid skin aging
Teeth and finger stains
Periodontal disease
Low libido
Impotence
Heartburn
Peptic ulcers
Hiatal hernia
Allergies
Rhinitis/sinusitis

Lowered immunity
Other infections
Blood disorders
Nutrient deficiencies
Acute bronchitis
Chronic bronchitis
Emphysema
Increased cholesterol
Atherosclerosis
Hypertension
Angina pectoris
Circulation
   insufficiency
Heart and artery
   disease
Heart attacks and
   strokes
Varicose veins
Osteoporosis

Cancers:
   Lung
   Mouth and tongue
   Larynx
   Esophagus
   Bladder
   Cervix
   Pancreas
   Kidney
Surgical complications
Increased pregnancy
   risks
Increased infant
   mortality
Burns from fires
Increased caffeine use
Increased alcohol use
More job and home
   changes
Higher insurance and
   medical fees

friends or with alcohol—and usually only during certain times of the day or week. Next are those who smoke in response to stress, mainly at work, and who may stop and start periodically. These two types usually find it easier to cut down or stop. Those who are all-day-long smokers have a strong physical and psychological addiction and going more than an hour without nicotine brings on withdrawal symptoms such as irritability, anxiety, or headaches. Often, the psychological factors are more intense than the physical ones. Consuming two or more packs a day indicates a strong addiction; medical and psychological support will likely be necessary to quit successfully. Specialized smoking-cessation programs are often useful.

Contrary to current marketing hype about low-tar, low-nicotine cigarettes, there are no safe smoking options. Some of the newer "lights" may be even worse than regular cigarettes because users inhale more deeply and smoke more frequently to satisfy nicotine needs. More carbon monoxide, hydrogen cyanide, and nitrogen gases are consumed with many of these low-nicotine cigarettes, and this can increase the oxygen deficit, heart disease, and lung damage associated with smoking.

What smokers really need are high-nicotine, low-tar cigarettes, so that they will smoke less for the same amount of nicotine (this is what a nicotine patch does, for example). Even better would be a way to get nicotine into the blood without smoke at all. Nicotine gum works well, and nicotine skin patches are now used in smoking-cessation programs. Nicotine oral inhalers and nasal sprays are also being used in conjunction with smoking cessation programs.[18] There are also nicotine lozenges and sublingual tablets to help satisfy the craving. The antidepressant drug Wellbutrin is also being used successfully in helping people control their cravings for and their addiction to nicotine as well as kick their habit over time.[19]

All of these options will still be moderately hazardous to our health, but much less so than smoking. They will also get rid of the primary and secondary risks due to smoke and smoke-borne chemicals.

Among current U.S. adult smokers, 70 percent report they want to quit and millions have attempted to quit.[20] In 2008, an estimated 48 million adults (aged eighteen years or older) were former smokers while 45 percent of adult smokers (nearly 21 million people) tried to stop smoking during the previous twelve months.[21] The number of heavy smokers in the United States continues to drop each year; when

we do this, we immediately begin to lower our potential for disease.[22]

Cigarette smoking puts us at risk through three primary degenerative disease–producing effects:

1. Irritation and inflammation

2. Free-radical generation

3. Allergy-addiction

Respiratory and cardiovascular diseases are the greatest and deadliest long-term consequences of smoking. The following list includes many of the nicotine issues:

- Cardiovascular disease (CVD), or the process of atherosclerosis, develops from the inflammatory effects and cholesterol-increasing effects of nicotine on the circulatory system.

- The carbon monoxide in inhaled smoke reduces the delivery of oxygen to our cells.

- Reduced oxygen levels cause our body to produce more red blood cells (polycythemia).

- CVD is primarily responsible for the decreased life expectancy associated with smoking, even more so than lung cancer, which usually only arises after twenty to thirty years of use, while circulatory effects start immediately.

- The three primary contributors to CVD are smoking, hypertension, and high cholesterol; smoking increases the incidence of the latter twofold.

- Nicotine lowers the level of protective HDL cholesterol.

- Decreased circulation and increased peripheral vascular resistance cause the heart to work harder with every beat and contributes to elevated blood pressure.

- Increased platelet aggregation leads to strokes and heart attacks. Smokers are three times more likely than nonsmokers to suffer heart attacks, mostly of the artery-spasm type. The pre-heart attack propensity to angina pectoris is also higher. Nicotine (and other agents in smoke) increases the incidence of arrhythmias (irregular heartbeat).

- Cerebral aneurysm (ballooning of the artery wall) is another risk that may be fatal.

- Peripheral vascular disease (disease of the arteries in the extremities) may manifest as intermittent claudication (pain in the legs when walking), as the poor circulation caused by atherosclerosis and vasoconstriction reduces oxygen delivery to the muscles.

- Buerger's disease is an arterial disease that may be caused by a hypersensitivity or an allergy to tobacco. The inflammation and scarring of the arteries in the arms and legs may even lead to amputation.

- Chronic inhalation of tobacco smoke eventually destroys lung tissue through a process of irritation, inflammation, and scarring.

- A higher than average incidence of respiratory infections, including colds and flus, bronchitis, and sinusitis, occurs with smoking. Cigarette smoke causes temporary paralysis of the cilia (fine hairs on the mucous linings that protect the deeper tissues from microorganisms and other foreign materials). The thinning and drying of the mucus itself dries and irritates the bronchial tubes.

- Chronic bronchitis, one form of chronic obstructive pulmonary disease (COPD), results from long-term irritation, loss of mucus protection, and recurrent infection, with a subsequent loss of lung capacity and function. This limitation in respiratory function occurs very near the onset of smoking. When smoking is stopped, much of the function returns, unless there is lung tissue scarring, which is irreversible.

- Smoking generally decreases lung capacity and endurance and with it, the desire or ability to exercise. Emphysema, another form of COPD, results from progressive scarring and loss of lung elasticity.

- Male smokers are twenty-three times more likely to contract lung cancer than nonsmokers, while female smokers are thirteen times more likely than nonsmokers to get lung cancer.[23] Some data suggest a slightly smaller likelihood of ten to twenty times that a smoker will develop lung cancer.[24] Yet, about 10 percent to 15 percent of people, especially women, with lung cancer have never smoked.[25] Thus, other factors are still to be determined. These cancer rates are even further increased with occupational exposure to agents such as asbestos, coal, textiles, and other chemicals. With heavy alcohol use, smokers may increase their risk of lung cancer.[26]

- Many other cancer rates are also higher for smokers, particularly for heavy alcohol-drinking smokers who are exposed to other carcinogenic chemicals, such as asbestos.

- Allergy-addiction symptoms may appear when smoking is first begun and then decrease with continued smoking.

- Increased atherosclerosis and subsequent decrease in blood circulation to the brain lead to memory loss and thinking problems, as well as early dementia. Recent research shows that heavy smokers in midlife have a very high risk of Alzheimer's disease.[27]

- Poor oxygen delivery to the skin and general dehydration of the tissues caused by smoking ages the skin and increases the number of deep wrinkles.

- Worldwide reports show how smoking affects sexuality and reproduction. In men, smoking has been shown to lower sperm counts and reproductive ability. Smoking may also cause genetic mutation, as there appears to be a slightly higher incidence of congenital malformations in the offspring of men who smoke.

SMOKERS AT HIGHER RISK

Pregnant women

Nursing mothers

Diabetics

Women using birth control pills

People with family history of heart disease

People with high blood pressure

People with high cholesterol

Heavy smokers

Obese people

Very thin people

Alcoholics or alcohol abusers (daily users)

People with existing smoker's disease

People who work with toxic chemicals

People having surgery

Ulcer patients

- In women who smoke, there are clearly more miscarriages and babies with lower birth weights.

- Smoking also increases the incidence of stillbirths, congenital malformations, and early infant deaths.

- Smoking around newborns and infants increases their susceptibility to many diseases, particularly colds, ear infections, bronchitis, and pneumonia.

- Women are at risk for all of the problems described in this list, but are particularly vulnerable if they are using birth control pills. For example, women who smoke and use the pill are twenty-five times more likely to suffer a heart attack than women who do neither.

- Although snuff and chewing tobacco are less toxic, chronic use of nicotine affects the circulatory system. There are currently more than 10 million chewers addicted to nicotine; even though they are not exposed to smoke, they still have the negative cardiovascular effects and a higher incidence of mouth, tongue, and throat cancers than nonsmokers do. The smoke from cigars and pipes is not usually inhaled (some is), so less nicotine and tars are absorbed with their use, although local irritation is possible.

- Smoking reduces appetite and taste for food, thus interfering with good nutrition.

- The risk of developing osteoporosis is increased with smoking due to poor calcium utilization.

- Smokers have a higher incidence of heartburn, hiatal hernia, and peptic ulcers.

- With smoking there is an increased risk of fire.

WHAT ABOUT SECONDHAND SMOKE?

Secondhand smoke has become a human rights issue in the last couple of decades as people feel that it is a violation of their right to breathe clean air. Secondary smoke is potentially more dangerous than mainstream smoke because it is not filtered. Of the sixteen or so poisons that arise from burning cigarettes, most are known carcinogens. Much of the ammonia, formaldehyde, acetaldehyde, formic acid, phenol, hydrogen sulfide, acetonitrile, and methyl chloride are filtered through the cigarette filters and are more concentrated in the smoke that wafts into the air. This is the smoke that passive, involuntary smokers inhale. Carbon monoxide levels in secondhand smokers are more than 50 percent higher than in those not exposed to cigarette smoke and often exceed carbon monoxide levels of light firsthand smokers.

A review of more than two thousand studies regarding secondhand smoke suggests that it increases the incidence of most of the diseases associated with smoking. Children of smokers have increased incidence of respiratory infections, ear infections, and lower lung function than do children of nonsmokers. Secondhand smoke increases the risk of COPD, heart disease, and lung cancer. In fact, an estimated three thousand cases of lung cancers per year are caused by secondhand smoke. It has been found that nonsmoking wives of male smokers have life expectancies that are four years shorter than those of nonsmoking wives of nonsmokers.

HOW DO WE DETOXIFY FROM NICOTINE?

A good air filter is an important preventive measure and can be very effective in removing toxins from the air; a basic multiple vitamin-mineral and antioxidant formula will help protect us internally. The daily program should include at least the nutrients in the chart on page 157.

Dietary Recommendations

No support program for smokers will be as effective as ceasing to smoke completely and working to regain lost health. A wholesome diet and nutritional supplements can help protect us from some of the effects of smoking; however, even the best program cannot offer immunity. There is a tendency for poor dietary habits to accompany the destructive smoking habit. Many smokers tend to eat more meats and fatty, fried, and refined foods than nonsmokers do, although there are smoking vegetarians, smoking exercise fanatics, and smoking health enthusiasts.

This plan, with adequate fruits, vegetables, and whole grains, will help replenish the protective antioxidant nutrients such as vitamins C, E, and A, beta-carotene, and selenium. In addition, raw seeds and nuts, legumes, sprouts, and other proteins should be consumed. Water is essential to balance out the drying effects of smoking and its toxicity. Caffeine also increases the need for water, because it is dehydrating. A daily intake of 2 to 3 quarts of liquid is suggested, depending on how many high-water-content fruits, vegetables, salads, juices, and soups are consumed. Because smoking usually generates an acidic condition in the body, I recommend following the Detox Diet plan. A high-fiber diet helps detoxification by maintaining bowel function.

The nutritional strategy for smokers is to increase the intake of wholesome foods—fruits, vegetables, and whole grains—and decrease the intake of fats and fried foods, cured or pickled products, food additives, and alcohol. The increased blood and tissue alkalinity that results from this diet helps reduce the craving for smoking, as shown by studies and my patients' reports.

An alkaline diet is not necessarily needed over an entire lifetime, although generally, it is preferable to an acidic diet.

STOP-SMOKING DIET

Increase Alkaline Foods
Examples:

Fruits	Figs
Vegetables	Raisins
Greens	Carrots
Lima beans	Celery
Millet	Almonds

Reduce Acid Foods
Examples:

Meats	Beef
Sugar	Chicken
Wheat	Eggs
Bread	Milk
Baked goods	Cheese

SMOKER'S SIMPLE NUTRIENT PLAN

Vitamin C	1,000 to 2,000 mg, up to 6 to 8 g daily
Mixed carotenoids*	15,000 to 25,000 IU, up to 50,000 IU
Vitamin A	5,000 to 10,000 IU
Zinc	15 to 30 mg
Selenium	200 mcg
Vitamin E	400 IU
L-tryptophan**	500 to 1,000 mg

* Although beta-carotene did not fare well in past studies for smokers when used solely, I believe its action within a complete antioxidant formula is still warranted based on a number of other positive studies. Here, the mixed carotenoids are likely more helpful than beta-carotene alone.

** L-tryptophan has been found to not only curb withdrawal symptoms in people getting off cigarettes but also lessen depression and support sleep when taken at night.

During cigarette withdrawal, a vegetarian or raw food diet may sufficiently reduce nicotine craving and can be used for three to six weeks to aid in the detoxification process. Fasting has also been employed by some smokers to help eliminate their habit. It is a means of rapid transition, but it is also somewhat intense. A juice fast under medical supervision might best be used with the very determined person or with the overweight or hypertensive smoker.

Several weeks of the Detox Diet (page 68) can be very effective at clearing the smoker's desire, habit, and chemicals from the body. Over a longer time, a vegetarian diet high in chlorophyllic (green) vegetables and sprouts, grains, fruits, and liquids such as water, juices, soups, and herbal teas is preferable. The raw foods diet is similar, but includes more seeds and nuts. Eating raw, unsalted sunflower seeds (or carrot or celery sticks) can help replace that hand-to-mouth habit we reinforce when we smoke. However, we must be careful not to replace nicotine addiction with new food addictions, but with better exercise and breathing habits, gardening, massage, and so on.

The diet for detoxification is low in fat and high in fiber, which helps keep energy levels high and the gut cleansed. Raw and vegetarian foods help with both. The diet includes several salads of leafy greens daily, and some fruit, vegetable, nut, or seed snacks. Some of the high-protein algaes such as spirulina, blue-green algae, and chlorella also help during withdrawal and detox.

Supplements

To support body alkalization during smoking cessation, take sodium or potassium bicarbonate tablets; take one to two during each period of craving up to a total of five or six tablets daily. A general multiple vitamin-mineral with additional antioxidant nutrients is an important part of the smoker's program (see pages 157 and 164 for all dosages). The antioxidants help reduce the toxicity of smoke in primary and secondary smokers and also help lessen free-radical irritation during the detox period.

Vitamin E helps stabilize cell membranes, protecting them and the tissue membranes from free radicals and chemical irritations. Selenium, as sodium selenite or selenomethionine, supports vitamin E and also reduces cancer potential. Selenium also lessens sensitivity to cadmium. Vitamin A reduces cancer risk and supports tissue health; beta-carotene may still offer some protection against the problems of smoking when used with other antioxidants.

Smokers need regular vitamin C intake to help neutralize the toxins and compensate for reduced absorption. (*Note:* Since both vitamin C and niacin are mild acids, they may aggravate any irritations in the gut, and thus may increase ulcer risk as well as nicotine cravings in smokers. If vitamin C or niacin is used in higher amounts, added alkaline salts such as the bicarbonates or calcium-magnesium ascorbates may be used.) Extra zinc, 30 to 60 mg a day, like vitamin A, helps protect the tissues and mucous membranes and reduces cadmium toxicity and absorption. If higher levels of zinc (over 60 mg daily) are taken, supplement with 3 to 4 mg of copper and 5 to 10 mg of manganese.

We need the support of the **B vitamins**, particularly thiamine (B_1), pyridoxine (B_6), and cobalamin (B_{12}). B_{12} is thought to help decrease the cellular damage caused by tars and nicotine. Niacin (B_3) helps open up constricted circulation. It also helps lower cholesterol and triglyceride levels, which may reduce the risk of atherosclerosis. Pantothenic acid (B_5) may slow skin aging and the effects of stress. Folic acid should be taken in higher amounts—even 1 to 2 mg or more are well tolerated—and offers some cardiovascular protection. Coenzyme Q10 can be helpful, and extra choline supports the brain and memory. Magnesium and molybdenum are also needed in higher amounts than usual.

N-acetyl-cysteine (NAC), along with thiamine and vitamin C, protect the lungs from acetaldehyde generated by smoking, and helps reduce smoker's cough. This can be taken in the form of 250 mg of NAC two or three times daily. Glutathione, formed from L-cysteine, is part of the protective antioxidant enzyme system. Heavy smokers might use 250 to 500 mg of glutathione, up to 1,500 mg (usually 500 to 750 mg) of NAC, with 5 to 6 g of vitamin C, 150 mg of thiamine, the total B vitamins, and a balanced amino acid formula daily.

To prevent significant weight gain during and following smoking cessation, it is very important to be aware of our eating habits. Because smoking reduces appetite and increases metabolism, it is natural to want to eat more when not smoking. Replace smoking with exercise or new activities. Smokers seem to crave and eat fewer sweets than nonsmokers; however, this changes with smoking cessation as the taste buds come alive again. Over half of ex-smokers will gain weight when they stop smoking, and this is even more common in heavier-use smokers. If weight gain is undesirable (many smokers are underweight and should gain weight), a weight-control diet should be instituted as smoking is stopped. The alkaline, high-fiber, low-fat diet is helpful in maintaining weight. Another amino acid, L-phenylalanine, can help reduce the appetite if taken before meals in amounts of 250 to 500 mg. However, its mild tendency to raise blood pressure should be taken into consideration. (This may be countered by the tendency of the blood pressure to drop somewhat with smoking cessation.) More choline may improve fat utilization and maintain weight, as may the amino acid L-carnitine. Regular exercise and plenty of fresh air are also part of the plan.

The level of nicotine addiction is based upon daily amounts and total number of years smoking, and will determine the ease of cessation. If you light up first thing in the morning or if you smoke more than two packs a day, it may be harder for you to stop than for lighter smokers.

PLAN TO STOP SMOKING

I have found that it is helpful for people to compose a plan and schedule of cessation dates and stages of nonsmoking before quitting, and document the reasons for doing so. Pick a low-stress time to stop, such as during vacation or just after sick leave from work or school. New Year's Day, your birthday, or national stop smoking days are other good choices. Keep notes of your process and feelings. Get to know yourself better through this process; many smokers release a lot of energy and excitement as they quit, so use this to construct new and better habits in all areas of your life.

There are many different cessation plans. The simplest way is just to make a firm decision and go cold turkey—there is no back and forth, no doubt; the decision is made. But only about 4 to 7 percent of people are able to quit smoking on any given attempt without medicines or other help.[28] Medical studies have reported that about 25 percent of smokers who use medicines can stay smoke-free for more than six months. Counseling and other types of emotional support can boost success rates higher than medicines alone. There is also early evidence that combining some medicines may work better than using a single drug.[29]

Withdrawal is not easy. The first three days to a week can be very difficult; for some people, the struggle may last for months. Usually, the first twelve to twenty-four hours are the peak of withdrawal, when symptoms may appear and when cigarette craving is almost omnipresent. During withdrawal, take one gram of vitamin C (as a mineral ascorbate—calcium or magnesium—to reduce acidity) every one or two hours. This may help reduce nicotine cravings.

If you just cannot give up nicotine, there are other ways to get rid of cigarettes. Though not ideal, they are at least one step better than smoking. Nicorette, a nicotine gum, is now available without prescription and can be a very useful transitional tool; nicotine patches in varying strengths are also being used.

The American Lung Association and the federal government endorse nicotine replacement therapy (NRT). Hundreds of clinical trials (including a National Institutes of Health–supported study involving people who used nicotine gum for five years) and extensive use over a number of years have proven the safety and efficacy of NRT products when used as directed. In direct contrast, tobacco smoke contains more than forty known carcinogens, plus many other toxins, such as carbon monoxide, arsenic, and ammonia, as well as substances that can trigger heart disease, emphysema, and many other life-threatening diseases.

Leading experts in the field of smoking control agree that NRT products have a crucial role to play in helping reduce the devastating toll of disease caused by tobacco dependence. One concern is, however, that people will abuse these patches and gum, using them while also smoking.

METHODS FOR QUITTING

"Cold turkey"
Behavioral modification
Smoking cessation aids:
    Nicotine gum
    Nicotine inhalers
    Nicotine patches
    Bupropion (Wellbutrin)
    Nicotine nasal spray

We suggest only using NRTs as directed by the manufacturer. Call your local American Cancer Society, American Lung Association at 1-800-LUNG-USA (1-800-586-4872) or visit their website at www.lungusa.org to find out more about how to stop smoking for good.

Both nicotine gum and patches are commonly used methods for smoking cessation that support nicotine addiction without harmful smoke chemicals. They reduce withdrawal symptoms, and research suggests a better long-term quitting percentage for those using them. They are, however, temporary aids. These substances may cause nausea, lightheadedness, hiccups, and muscle tension or jaw aches from chewing. They do, however, immediately help people stop smoking, because most of the nicotine craving is satisfied. The smoking response must still be addressed, and the former smoker should be off the gum or patches within a couple of months, or sometimes longer. (Patches may even need to be used for a year to be successful.) Research suggests that people with ulcers or cardiovascular disease should avoid these methods, as should pregnant women. "Smokeless" cigarettes can be used for withdrawal and transition as well.

If none of these methods alone is successful for you, there are behavioral and supportive therapies to help stay smoke-free. Check the package insert of any nicotine product you are using to see if the manufacturer provides free telephone-based counseling. Working to smoke fewer cigarettes daily is a common practice, but

generally ten per day is needed to satisfy the nicotine habit. You might also try taking fewer puffs per cigarette or smoking just the first half of each, where the least amounts of tars and chemicals are concentrated. Filters and cigarette holders also decrease the amount of toxic elements inhaled. There are devices that place tiny holes in cigarette filters to allow dilution of smoke with outside air. You might also try changing brands to lower-tar, higher-nicotine cigarettes or using brands you do not like. For anyone who smokes, avoid chemically treated cigarettes and using natural, untreated tobacco and untreated paper.

STOP SMOKING BREW

3 parts dandelion root

1 part valerian root

3 parts lemongrass

2 parts red clover leaf

2 parts mullein leaf

2 parts alfalfa

2 parts raspberry leaf

2 parts peppermint

1 part catnip

Simmer the dandelion and valerian in water for 10 minutes, then pour into a pot containing the other herbs and steep for 15 minutes. Drink 1 cup several times daily or as needed for cravings.

SUGGESTIONS FOR SMOKING CESSATION

- **Cut down on other addictive substances,** such as caffeine, sugar, and alcohol, all of which can increase the desire to smoke.

- **Get another smoker to stop** with you or, even better, get an ex-smoker to support you while you stop.

- **Tell empathetic friends** or family and ask for their support—that is, go public with your plan to stop.

- **Stay busy** to prevent boredom and to keep your mind off smoking.

- **Exercise regularly** to decrease withdrawal, increase motivation, and increase relaxation. Include your favorite aerobic sport and try to do it outdoors.

- If you don't enjoy **vigorous exercise,** consider a yoga class, swimming, or low-impact aerobics.

- **Create rewards** for being successful and implement them daily.

- **Get plenty of rest.**

- **Drink fluids** and use water for therapy by taking showers, baths, saunas, or hot tubs, or by going swimming.

- **Change daily patterns** to avoid stimulating old smoking conditioning. This may include staying away from bars, alcohol, and coffee, avoiding friends who smoke, not receiving or making phone calls at specific locations in which you usually smoked, and getting up and doing something right after a meal.

- **Learn and practice relaxation** and breathing techniques.

- **Practice visualization.**

- **Keep a positive attitude** toward health and life.

- **Get health treatments,** such as massage or teeth cleaning to remove cigarette stains.

- **Find temporary oral substitutes** to deal with psychological ties to smoking. Oral fixation substitutes could include munchies such as vegetable sticks (carrot, celery, zucchini), apples, nuts, popcorn, sunflower seeds (unsalted) in shells, sugarless hard candies or nonedible substitutes such as gum, or chewing or sucking on ice cubes, toothpicks, licorice sticks, or drinking straws.

- **If cravings arise,** find ways to deal with them. Take a short break, a walk, or a shower; drink tea; or do things with your hands, such as sketching or doodling, working a crossword puzzle, or making a shopping list. Breathe and relax, and be thankful you are not smoking.

I have found that it is helpful for people to compose a plan and schedule of cessation dates and stages of nonsmoking before quitting, and document your reasons for doing so. Pick a low-stress time to stop, such as during vacation or just after sick leave from work or school. New Year's Day, your birthday, or national stop smoking days are other good choices. Keep notes of your process and feelings. Get to know yourself better through this process; many smokers release a lot of energy and excitement as they quit, so use this to construct new and better habits in all areas of your life.

MAKE THE COMMITMENT TO STOP

When you quit, make a commitment. If you have trouble doing this, find someone with lung cancer or emphysema to talk with. Know your cigarette triggers and work to defuse them. Get rid of ashtrays, clean your teeth and your home, and make your life a nonsmoking zone. Take extra special care of yourself with good foods, pure drinking water, hot baths or showers, exercise, and massage. Reward yourself with a trip to the mountains, an afternoon off at the movies, or a day at a spa or beauty salon. Get your mind off yourself by getting involved with others: volunteer, coach or play on a softball team, or organize a fund-raiser for your community. Learn a new language or musical instrument; try gardening or a new sport.

Breathe fresh air, walk, and get your heart beating harder.

It is crucial for people who stop smoking to become highly skilled at handling stress. Most people who start smoking again do so when they are under increased stress. Relaxation tapes, classes, and counseling can help. Stress-reduction plans and exercises—both mental and physical—are also helpful. Use your own support system at these times. These plans for exercise and stress management are best initiated before smoking cessation, so the necessary tools will already be in place. Also, regular exercise and relaxation may reinforce the need to cut down or quit. In fact, regular exercise offers many of the same feelings smokers get from nicotine, such as an "up" feeling, confidence, and a greater ability to relax and concentrate.

It is important to maintain a positive attitude and use affirmations such as "I am not a smoker" or "Stopping smoking is a great benefit to my health." Or try this: "I am not a cigarette or an ashtray. I am not supporting the greedy cigarette industry; they don't pay my health insurance." Write them down and post them in specific areas as reminders. Many ex-smokers use negative imagery to stay away from cigarettes. They think of lung damage, heart disease, wrinkled skin, or limited activity whenever they feel the urge to smoke. If we visualize these negative images when we take a deep breath and hold it, the negative feedback we feel while oxygen levels are decreasing and carbon dioxide levels are rising will help

NICOTINE NUTRIENT PROGRAM

Water	2 to 3 qt	Chromium	200 to 500 mcg
Fat (low)	30 to 50 g	Copper	2 to 4 mg
Fiber	15 to 45 g	Iodine	150 to 250 mcg
Vitamin A	5,000 to 10,000 IU	Iron*	women: 15 to 30 mg men: 5 to 10 mg
Mixed carotenoids	20,000 to 40,000 IU	Magnesium	500 to 1,000 mg
Vitamin D	400 to 2,000 IU	Manganese	5 to 10 mg
Vitamin E	400 to 800 IU	Molybdenum	300 to 600 mcg
Vitamin K	100 to 300 mcg	Potassium	200 to 500 mg
Thiamine (B₁)	100 to 200 mg	Selenium	200 to 400 mcg
Riboflavin (B₂)	50 to 100 mg	Silicon	50 to 150 mg
Niacinamide (B₃)	50 to 100 mg	Vanadium	150 to 300 mcg
Niacin (B₃)	100 to 1,000 mg	Zinc	30 to 75 mg
Pantothenic acid (B₅)	250 to 1,000 mg	Coenzyme Q10	50 to 100 mg
Pyridoxine (B₆), and/or	50 to 100 mg,	L-amino acids	1,000 to 2,000 mg
Pyridoxal-5-phosphate	25 to 75 mg	L-tryptophan**	500 mg at bed
Cobalamin (B₁₂)	200 to 1,000 mcg	L-cysteine (or NAC)	500 to 1,500 mg
Folic acid	800 to 2,000 mcg	Glutathione	250 to 500 mg
Biotin	200 to 500 mcg	Glycine	250 to 500 mg
Choline	500 to 1,000 mg	Omega-3 essential fatty acids or	4 to 6 capsules
PABA	500 to 1,000 mg	Flaxseed oil	2 to 3 teaspoons
Vitamin C	3 to 12 g		
Bioflavonoids	250 to 750 mg	**For Withdrawal and Detox:**	
Quercetin	400 mg	Garlic	3 to 6 capsules
Calcium	600 to 1,200 mg	Valerian root	4 to 6 capsules
		Lobelia leaf	1 to 2 capsules
		Carrot sticks	10 to 20

* Levels depend on the body's needs and blood loss.
** A study found that tryptophan supplements reduced withdrawal symptoms and helped people smoke fewer cigarettes when taken with a high-carbohydrate diet.

us stay off cigarettes. We should remind ourselves that we are grappling with a substance more addicting than heroin and scientifically designed to keep us involved as paying customers—then banish it! Even more important is visualizing the positive benefits, such as the new ability to taste and smell, better digestion, improved respiratory and circulatory functions, and the chance for a longer and healthier life. Increasing the love we have for ourselves as nonsmokers and continuing to see ourselves as nonsmokers are key. Every day we are not smoking, we are making progress toward improved health and better kissing!

Smoking certain herbs has been used to replace cigarettes temporarily or to treat bronchopulmonary problems. Mullein leaf is probably the most commonly used. Coltsfoot, yerba santa, sarsaparilla, and rosemary have also been smoked. Lobelia leaf, called "Indian tobacco," has been employed as a cigarette substitute because it acts and tastes a bit like tobacco. In China, other herbs are smoked to treat asthma and other respiratory problems. Ginseng leaf and other herbal cigarettes have been available. Smoking mugwort or catnip may help in relaxation; damiana is thought to have aphrodisiac properties; peppermint added to other blends gives a cool, menthol taste, and licorice adds a sweet flavor. Yet, realize that generally **inhaling any smoke is not great for our lungs.** Chewing licorice sticks replaces the oral habit and settles the system. Chewing calamus root is a nicotine

version of Antabuse. Garlic (taken orally, not smoked) is also helpful during the tobacco detox period.

A program that combines other supportive therapies, including acupuncture, counseling, hypnosis, and massage, with diet and supplements works wonderfully but can be time-consuming and costly. Consider adding one of these forms of support to your plan. There are a number of good smoking cessation programs available in most cities and often the cost commitment and group support add extra incentive. Avoid rapid smoking plans that make you sicker to get well, because the excessive nicotine you will ingest can be toxic. A desire to stop and the willpower to continue pursuing a nonsmoking lifestyle are at the heart of all successful programs.

The nutrient levels in the table on page 164 can be spread out in several portions throughout the day. Vitamin C can be used even more frequently. The dosages range from smoker's support (low) to complete nicotine withdrawal (high), with the three to six weeks of initial detoxification requiring a mid-range amount.

NICOTINE DETOX SUMMARY

1. **Eat an alkaline diet** of fruits, vegetables, and whole grains. Follow the Detox Diet, or try a vegetarian or raw foods diet during detox. Reduce acid foods and potential carcinogens, such as fats, food additives, and alcohol.

2. **Drink 2 to 3 quarts of pure water a day.**

3. **Keep fiber intake high** to support detoxification and colon function.

4. **Maintain vitamin levels** through supplementation (see previous page). If cravings are strong, take 1 gram of vitamin C every one to two hours.

5. Also, **take sodium or potassium bicarbonate** tablets to alkalinize your body—one for each occasion of craving, but not more than six daily.

6. **Use herbal supplements,** including herbal stop-smoking brews.

7. **Exercise,** especially in the fresh air, to oxygenate your body.

8. If you are having **real difficulty** staying away from cigarettes, consider the use of nicotine patches or gum to help your transition.

9. **Use acupuncture** or hypnosis to motivate you to stop and/or support you during withdrawal and detox.

10. **Ease detox** with relaxing therapies—hot baths or showers, saunas or hot tubs, swimming, and massage.

11. **Practice relaxation** and deep breathing. Get to know nature.

12. **Build a method of support** into your plan, including friends, family, and counseling. Stay busy and know that you are taking care of yourself, especially for the future.

13. **Find oral substitutes** for smoking. Change daily patterns to avoid smoking stimuli.

14. **Do a journal/tape** review of how and when you were first influenced to smoke. Evaluate the focus of your new and previous relationship to smoking.

Endnotes

1. www.cdc.gov/tobacco/data_statistics/fact_sheets/fast_facts.
2. "Smoking-Attributable Mortality, Years of Potential Life Lost, and Productivity Losses—United States, 2000–2004," *MMWR* 57, no. 45 (November 14, 2008); www.cdc.gov/tobacco/data_statistics/fact_sheets/health_effects/effects_cig_smoking.
3. Ibid.
4. Substance Abuse and Mental Health Administration, "Results from the 2009 National Survey on Drug Use and Health: National Findings Exit Notification." Rockville, MD: Office of Applied Studies, 2009.

5. 2006 Surgeon General's Report—The Health Consequences of Involuntary Exposure to Tobacco Smoke.

6. www.cdc.gov/chronicdisease/resources/publications/aag/osh.htm.

7. Ibid.

8. Ibid.

9. National Cancer Institute, "Cancer Trends Progress Report 2009/2010." http://progressreport.cancer.gov/doc_detail.asp?pid=1&did=2007&chid=71&coid=703&mid.

10. Centers for Disease Control and Prevention, "Vital Signs: Current Cigarette Smoking Among Adults Aged ≥ 18 Years—United States, 2009." *Morbidity and Mortality Weekly Report* 59, no. 35 (2010): 1135–40 (accessed January 14, 2011).

11. A. Ventura, D. G. Kirsch, M.E. McLaughlin, D.A. Tuveson, J. Grimm, L. Lintault, J. Newman, E.E. Reczek, R. Weissleder, and T. Jacks, "Restoration of p53 Function Leads to Tumour Regression In Vivo," *Nature* 445, no. 7128 (2007): 661–5.

12. Tom Ferguson, *The Smoker's Book of Health: How to Keep Yourself Healthier and Reduce Your Smoking* (New York: Putnam, 1987).

13. A.C. Parsons, M. Shraim, J. Inglis, P. Aveyard, and P. Hajek, "Interventions for Preventing Weight Gain After Smoking Cessation," *Cochrane Database of Systematic Reviews* 1 (January 2009); David F. Williamson et al., "Smoking Cessation and Severity of Weight Gain in a National Cohort," *New England Journal of Medicine* 324: (March 14, 1991): 739–45.

14. G.N. Connolly, H.R. Alpert, G.F. Wayne, and H. Koh, "Trends in Nicotine Yield in Smoke and Its Relationship with Design Characteristics Among Popular US Cigarette Brands, 1997–2005," *Tobacco Control* 16, no. 5 (October 2007): e5.

15. www.ejnet.org/dioxin/; and www.greenfacts.org/en/dioxins/l-2/dioxins-1.htm.

16. www.epa.gov/radiation/sources/tobacco.html.

17. Mark Fischetti, "Radiation Sources Range from Cigarettes to CT Scans: How Many Millisieverts Are You Getting?" *Scientific American* (May 2011). www.scientificamerican.com/article.cfm?id=graphic-science-radiation-exposure.

18. www.nlm.nih.gov/medlineplus/druginfo/meds/a606020.html.

19. P. Tonnesen, S. Tonstad, A. Hjalmarson, F. Lebargy, P.I. Van Spiegel, A. Hider, R. Sweet, and J. Townsend, "A Multicentre, Randomized, Double-Blind, Placebo-Controlled, 1-Year Study of Bupropion SR for Smoking Cessation," *Journal of Internal Medicine* 254, no. 2 (August 2003): 184–192; P. Wu, K. Wilson, P. Dimoulas, and E.J. Mills, "Effectiveness of Smoking Cessation Therapies: A Systematic Review and Meta-Analysis," *BMC Public Health* 6 (December 2006): 300–315.

20. www.cdc.gov/tobacco/data_statistics/fact_sheets/cessation/quitting.

21. Ibid.

22. John P. Pierce et al., "Prevalence of Heavy Smoking in California and the United States, 1965–2007," *Journal of the American Medical Association* 305, no. 11 (2011): 1106–12.

23. American Cancer Society, "Detailed Guide: Lung Cancer (Non-Small Cell). What Are the Key Statistics About Lung Cancer?" Updated 07/28/10. www.cancer.org/Cancer/LungCancer-Non-SmallCell/DetailedGuide/non-small-cell-lung-cancer-key-statistics.

24. www.cdc.gov/cancer/lung/basic_info/risk_factors.htm.

25. M. J. Thun, S.J. Henley, D. Burns, et al., "Lung Cancer Death Rates in Lifelong Nonsmokers," *Journal of the National Cancer Institute* 98 (2006): 691.

26. See note 24 above.

27. www.usatoday.com/yourlife/health/medical/alzheimers/2010-10-26-smokingAlz23_ST_N.htm.

28. American Cancer Society, "Guide to Quitting Smoking." www.cancer.org/Healthy/StayAwayfromTobacco/GuidetoQuittingSmoking/guide-to-quitting-smoking-success-rates.

29. www.smokefree.gov/tools.aspx.

CHAPTER TWELVE

Alcohol Detoxification

EVEN THOUGH ALCOHOL IS ENJOYED worldwide and has been used for thousands of years, its regular overconsumption poses a serious health hazard. The regular use of alcohol in the United States has been going down, yet the occasional weekend binge is going up.[1] As with caffeine, occasional or moderate use is often pleasurable and is no cause for concern except for people with allergic reactions to alcohol or diseases of the liver, gastrointestinal tract, kidneys, brain, or nervous system. Overconsumption depends on the frequency of use (as in tolerability) as well as body size, gender, and the ability to detoxify. (Some people are slow detoxifiers or have an enzyme deficiency such as associated with Gilbert's syndrome, which results in elevated blood bilirubin. These people may not tolerate much alcohol.) Habitual alcohol overconsumption, however, can lead to addiction, emotional problems, and a number of specific degenerative processes, including obesity, gastritis and ulcers, hepatitis, cirrhosis, pancreatitis, hypoglycemia and diabetes, gout, nerve and brain dysfunction, cancer, nutritional deficiencies, immune suppression, accidental injury, and death. Most people can handle periodic moderate use, but for many others, any alcohol can lead to significant problems.

Alcohol has some positive physiological effects.[2] It stimulates the appetite and conversation and relieves stress. It acts as a vasodilator, improving blood flow. Alcohol aids heart health by increasing good HDL cholesterol levels while also decreasing bad LDL cholesterol levels and thrombosis risk; however, it also raises total blood cholesterol and triglyceride levels. Small to moderate amounts (one or two drinks daily) may also lessen the progression of atherosclerosis and heart disease.

Most studies have shown a lower number of heart attacks in moderate drinkers compared with nondrinkers of the same age, possibly due to increased HDL cholesterol levels, blood vessel elasticity, and blood flow and reduced atherosclerosis. In fact, the current Dietary Guidelines for Americans 2010 and the CDC recognize moderate alcohol consumption as one of four key healthy lifestyle behaviors. Moderate consumption is one alcoholic drink for women and two for men.[3] It is also statistically relevant that moderate drinkers live longer than abstainers.[4] Higher amounts of alcohol, however, increase blood pressure and heart disease risk. More research is needed to understand the real link between alcohol (and the chemicals used) and heart disease before prescribing it as a preventive measure, though it is important to know that it is the overall lifestyle that is likely improving the health of moderate drinkers—typically they drink while sharing meals, for example. Certainly regular physical activity and nurturing personal relationships may be better health supporters and stress reducers than alcohol is.

Excessive drinking is defined by the CDC to include heavy drinking (for men more than two drinks per day; for women, more than one drink), binge drinking, or both. Binge drinking is defined as four (women) or five (men) or more drinks during a single occasion. Most people who binge drink are not alcoholics or alcohol dependent.[5]

As of 2009, 67 percent of adults in the United States drink alcohol.[6] Although there are slight yearly fluctuations, Gallup's polling of Americans show the percentage who say they drink alcohol has remained remarkably stable over the past seventy-one years. According to the Behavioral Risk Factor Surveillance System (BRFSS) survey, approximately 5 percent of the total population drank heavily, while 15 percent of the population binge drank in the thirty days prior to the survey.[7] About 11 million people reported heavy alcohol use. Men are more likely to be heavier drinkers and engage in riskier behaviors, such as careless driving and acting aggressively.[8] More than half of our population is composed of social drinkers (150 million). Social drinking and problem drinking (alcohol abuse) mean different things.[9] Not all abusers are alcohol dependent. Drinking too much and too often is abuse and problem drinking, but the person may not be an alcoholic. Treatment centers including the National Institute on Alcohol Abuse and Alcoholism (NIAAA) have a **CAGE system** to help determine whether you are a problem drinker. If you feel that alcohol is a problem for you, they ask you to consider the **following four questions:**

- Have you ever felt you should **C**ut down on your drinking?

- Have people **A**nnoyed you by criticizing your drinking?

- Have you ever felt **G**uilty about your drinking?

- Do you ever need an **E**ye opener—a drink first thing in the morning—to steady your nerves or get rid of a hangover?

One yes answer suggests alcohol is a problem. Alcoholism occurs when one becomes physically dependent upon alcohol, and is now considered a disease by the American Medical Association. To my patients, I suggest that if they drink every day, they should consider it a problem and take a break to assess the true nature of their relationship to alcohol.

Alcohol is a particularly big concern for our youth. In fact, alcohol is the most commonly used and abused drug among youth in the United States, more than tobacco and illicit drugs.[10] More and more children are trying alcohol, and in 2008 the National Survey on Drug Use and Health reported that 28 percent of Americans aged twelve to twenty years drank alcohol and 19 percent reported binge drinking.[11] A 2009 survey reported that 37 percent of eighth graders and 72 percent of twelfth graders had tried alcohol.[12] Another alarming fact is that young people who start drinking before age fifteen are five times more likely to develop alcohol dependence or abuse later in life than those who begin drinking at or after age twenty-one.[13]

Many approaches have been developed to help the problem drinker cut back or stop drinking altogether. The type of treatment reflects whether alcoholism is viewed as a disease or as a social issue, or both. An overall program includes alcohol detoxification (usually with the help of pharmaceuticals) followed by a combination of supportive therapy, attendance at self-help groups such as Alcoholics Anonymous, and ongoing development of coping mechanisms.[14]

The costs of alcohol abuse to human lives and the economy are enormous. According to the latest reports gathered by the NIAAA, alcohol abuse in the United States is responsible for $134 billion in lost productivity every year, plus $26 billion for health-care costs and $36 billion in crime and welfare costs.[15]

Yearly health-care expenses for treating alcohol-related illnesses include more than $7 billion spent in direct treatment and $19 billion spent on the treatment of medical consequences. Alcohol-related vehicle crashes cost the country more than $15 billion a year, while the criminal justice system spends more than $6 billion on alcohol-related crime.

EMPTY CALORIES MEAN INSUFFICIENT NUTRITION

Alcohol is a source of empty calories; it contains 7 calories of them per gram, almost double the calories found in regular carbohydrates and protein (4 calories per gram each, while a gram of fat is 9 calories). The typical 12-ounce glass of beer contains

149 calories; a 1-ounce serving of distilled spirits (gin, bourbon, brandy) contains 65 calories, and a 4-ounce glass of wine has about 80 calories. The average social drinker consumes 5 to 10 percent of his or her calories from alcohol, while heavy drinkers may consume more than 50 percent in place of real nutrition. Because alcohol is often replacing regular nutrition in the heavy drinker, that person receives decreased amounts of essential vitamins, minerals, and other nutrients, causing deficiencies over time. In addition, the alcohol molecule is so small and easy to absorb that it gets assimilated before other foods, directly entering the bloodstream for a quick effect. Beer, wine, and mixed drinks cause rapid fluctuations in blood sugar with accompanying mood swings. How quickly the alcohol is metabolized depends on whether it is taken with food or not. On an empty stomach, alcohol goes into the bloodstream quickly, while it may take several hours to be metabolized after eating a fatty meal.

The liver is the only organ that metabolizes alcohol, either converting it into sugars for energy or storing it as fat when there is excess consumption. When stored as fat, alcohol acts as a liver irritant and can eventually lead to cirrhosis or scarring of the liver tissue. About 5 percent of ingested alcohol is eliminated through sweat, urine, and breath.

Many people think of alcohol as a stimulant because it reduces inhibitions and, in small amounts, seems to ease and enhance social interactions. It is actually a sedative that depresses the central nervous system. The effects can be pleasantly tranquilizing at first. However, with continued consumption the calming effect deteriorates into mental and physical numbness, hampering our reflexes, coordination, and judgment. This is why there are so many alcohol-related accidents while walking, bicycling, and driving.

Despite all these problems, alcohol is rooted in our culture. For centuries, alcohol was used as an anesthetic to treat physical pain. Nowadays it is used to anesthetize emotional pain. Alcohol abuse and alcoholism are clearly diseases that involve genetics, social/cultural values, and environmental influences and that have emotional consequences. It is possible that alcohol may involve an enzyme deficiency or be linked to a deficiency or improper function of chromium (a trace mineral related to blood sugar metabolism). Research is beginning to show that several genetic markers are involved in the predisposition to alcohol abuse, including the genes that code the enzyme *alcohol dehyrogenase.*[16] Multiple factors, in addition to genetics, contribute to alcohol abuse in families.

Alcohol drinks can also be allergenic because of the grains, grapes, sugar, and yeast they may contain, producing both intestinal and cerebral symptoms. Alcoholism may even be an advanced food addiction in which the allergens themselves stimulate addiction. In such cases, withdrawal from the offending food initially produces uncomfortable

CALORIE CONTENT OF ALCOHOLIC BEVERAGES

Amount That Provides 0.6 oz of Alcohol*	Type of Beverage	Calories
1 oz	100- or 110-proof liquor	80
1½ oz	80-proof liquor	90 to 110
5 oz	8 to 10% wine (dry, white)	100
4 oz	12 to 14% wine (dry, red)	95
3 oz	17 to 20% wine (sherry, port)	80
3 oz	18% dessert wine	140
8 oz	6 to 7% dark beer (stout, porter)	150
12 oz	4.5% regular beer	150
12 oz	light beer	90
6 oz	mixed drinks (juices, sodas, sweeteners)	100 to 250

* In the United States, a standard drink is any drink that contains 0.6 ounces (13.7 grams or 1.2 tablespoons) of pure alcohol. Generally, this amount of pure alcohol is found in 12 ounces of regular beer, 8 ounces of malt liquor, 5 ounces of wine, and 1.5 ounces of 80-proof distilled spirits or liquor, such as gin, rum, vodka, and whiskey.

psychological and physical symptoms. Alcohol products are also problematic for people with a yeast overgrowth in the body (especially intestines), as they feed the yeast and stimulate its growth. Furthermore, many people react to various chemicals, such as sulfites, which are used in producing wine and beer.

It has been suggested that alcohol is a viable source of nourishment. Wine does contain vitamin C from grape or rice juice, yet it also contains 9 to 12 percent alcohol (empty calories). In sherry and port wine, alcohol content may be as high as 12 to 18 percent. Beer and ale contain B vitamins and minerals from the cereal grains and yeast, with a range from 3 to 6 percent alcohol. Alcohol distillates or spirits such as gin, vodka, rum, and whiskey are also made from grain products. These range from 35 to 50 percent alcohol—that is, 70 to 100 proof. In reality, none of these beverages is very nourishing when calorie levels are compared with nutrient levels.

RISKS OF ALCOHOL

The risks associated with alcohol are directly related to the amount consumed, the gender and weight of the individual, and the time period over which it is used, although some people can be more sensitive to small amounts. High-risk use involves more than five drinks daily; moderate-risk use, three to five drinks daily; and low-risk, one or two. Social drinking of a few drinks a week offers minimal risk.

Those with diabetes, hypertension, or heart disease, and pregnant or nursing mothers, or those planning pregnancy, should not drink alcohol at all. People under the age of twenty-one, or those with blood sugar problems, liver disorders (especially hepatitis), ulcers and gastritis, viral diseases, yeast problems, mental confusion, fatigue, or hypersensitive reactions to alcoholic beverages should also avoid it.

Symptoms from drinking include dizziness, delayed reflexes, slowed mental function, memory loss, poor judgment, emotional outbursts, aggressive behavior, lack of coordination, and loss of consciousness. **Symptoms of hangover** include mouth dryness, thirst, headache, throbbing temples, nausea, vomiting, stomach upset, fatigue, and dizziness. Alcohol dehydrates the cells, removes fluid from the blood, swells the cranial arteries, and irritates the gastrointestinal tract. Hangovers are more common with stronger, distilled alcohol drinks but can still occur with red and white wines, champagne, and beer.

Symptoms of withdrawal include alcohol craving, nausea, vomiting, gastrointestinal upset, abdominal cramps, dehydration, anorexia, fatigue, headache, anxiety, irritability, dizziness, fevers, chills, depression, insomnia, tremors, weakness, hallucinations, and seizures.

Drinking can put us at risk of inadvertently harming ourselves or others. Alcohol is involved in the more than 25,000 auto accident deaths yearly. About 20 percent of home accidental deaths are attributed to alcohol plus alcohol-related domestic violence.

Ninety-five percent of alcohol consumed must be metabolized in the liver, possibly taking precedence over other functions. Fat metabolism slows and fat builds up in the liver. Because alcohol converts into fat, obesity (especially abdominal obesity, the most dangerous area) also often occurs with high alcohol use. Chronic use can swell, scar, and shrink the liver, until only a small percentage is functional. Complications also include ascites (fluid buildup in the abdomen), hemorrhoids, varicose veins, and bleeding disorders. More serious liver diseases such as hepatitis and cirrhosis, when the liver becomes inflamed or enlarged (and scarred and less functional), are also the result of chronic alcohol use. Usually more than half the liver must be destroyed before its work is significantly impaired (but it can regenerate if drinking is stopped).

Gastrointestinal disorders include gastritis, abdominal pain, eating difficulties, gastric ulcers, duodenal ulcers, deficiency of hydrochloric acid and digestive enzymes, "leaky gut" syndrome, esophagitis (irritation of the esophagus), varicose veins, pancreatitis, gallstones, and gallbladder disease.

Alcohol can cross the blood-brain barrier, destroying brain cells and causing brain damage and behavioral and psychological problems; nervous system disorders, including polyneuritis (nerve inflammations), premature senility, and encephalopathy (chronic degenerative brain syndrome) can also result from chronic alcohol use.

Although modest alcohol intake may, in fact, raise HDL cholesterol and protect against atherosclerosis, the effect of alcohol abuse on the heart and blood vessels is damaging and leads to cardiovascular diseases and dysfunctions. These include a decrease in heart function, heart muscle action, and electrical conductivity, congestive heart failure, cardiac arrythmias, and an enlarged heart.

Carbohydrate metabolism is affected by alcohol and can lead to hypoglycemia and diabetes. Alcohol is a simple sugar that is rapidly absorbed and has a tendency to weaken glucose tolerance with chronic use. Impaired glucose metabolism can cause mood swings, depression, emotional outbursts, and anxiety. Furthermore, increased calories from alcohol can lead to weight gain and increased body fat, resulting in obesity as alcohol converts into fat unless it is balanced by exercise and a good diet.

Nutritional deficiencies from alcohol use potentially include impaired absorption of nutrients, particularly B vitamins and minerals; liver impairment from reduced absorption of the fat-soluble vitamins A, D, E, and K; loss of nutrients like potassium and magnesium from alcohol's diuretic effect; reduced liver stores of alcohol-metabolizing vitamins B_1 and B_3; anemia due to deficiency of folic acid, vitamin B_{12}, and iron; increased risk of osteoporosis from low vitamin D and poor calcium absorption; lack of appetite, causing deficiencies in vitamin B_2, B_6, A, C, essential fatty acids, methionine, or really any nutrient that comes from a good and wholesome diet.

Alcohol increases levels of the liver enzyme that breaks down testosterone. In teenage boys who drink, the reduction of testosterone may delay sexual maturity. Alcohol's depressant effect on the nervous system can reduce sexual performance or cause impotence despite reduced inhibitions and increased desire.

Alcohol has been implicated in malignancies of the mouth, esophagus, pancreas, and breasts. Cigarette smoke and alcohol combined are thought to create ethyl nitrite, which is a strong mutagen. Other health problems include a red swollen nose, dilated blood vessels, gout, yeast vaginitis, premenstrual syndrome, and a suppressed immune system. Because alcohol crosses the placenta and enters fetal circulation, fetal alcohol syndrome results in undersized babies often with mental deficits due to brain damage. There is no safe level of alcohol intake—women who are pregnant should simply not drink! Regular alcohol use and abuse can create social problems in personal relationships and careers, and economic adversity in regard to lost work and medical costs.

ALCOHOLISM

The alcoholic is someone who has lost control over the drug. Research suggests that there is a genetic component to problem drinking. An intense biological craving for alcohol or the products from which it is made may be at the root, as might problems with blood sugar metabolism or allergy-addictions. The ability to easily stop drinking for a week or two at a time is a good sign. Remember, many people with a drinking problem deny that there is one. **Warning signs of alcoholism** include drinking alone, drinking in place of meals, drinking before social or business functions, drinking in the morning or late at night, missing work because of drinking, and periods of amnesia or blackouts. People who have these concerns should definitely seek help.

Once we've admitted that we need outside resources to deal with alcohol, it is important to get the support of our spouse or a friend. Clear the alcohol from all areas of life (home, work, car, and so on), and then see a physician or therapist. A medical check-up with laboratory testing may be in order. Some cases require tranquilizers during the first few days of withdrawal. In 2009 almost half a million people entered treatment centers for help with alcohol abuse; another 300,000 had secondary drug addictions as well.[17] Based on data from the National Institute on Alcohol Abuse and Alcoholism, about one-third of the people who entered treatment programs for alcohol abuse are in full recovery one year later.[18]

Psychological counseling, family therapy, Alcoholics Anonymous (AA), or religious/spiritual practices may also improve our motivation, self-image, and ability to create a new life. AA meetings continue the positive support for many recovering alcoholics. Avoiding negative influences such as old drinking buddies and exposure to alcohol is also helpful. Regular exercise is valuable, especially at the usual drinking time. In addition, weight training is an excellent way to work off stress and anger. Learning and practicing relaxation exercises can also be useful. Massage therapy promotes relaxation and self-love. Acupuncture is usually beneficial during withdrawal and detox, as it seems to reduce the stress from cravings and other symptoms that may reappear periodically after the initial detox process.

The amount of time it takes to detoxify from alcohol depends on the level of abuse, and it may take months or even years to completely clear its effects. Mild withdrawal symptoms include increased tension, headaches, and irritability for a few days. Medical care in a hospital setting is not uncommon for acute alcohol withdrawal, although this is usually necessary only for those who consume more than six to eight drinks daily.

If willpower is poor, drugs such as Antabuse (disulfiram), which produce terrible nausea and vomiting when alcohol is used, can be a powerful deterrent. Antabuse is usually fairly well tolerated for a short time, but it can have side effects on the cardiovascular system and psyche. Lithium therapy has recently been shown to reduce the urge to drink. For recovering alcoholics, I believe that it is imperative to avoid all alcohol for life, because the addictive potential never disappears. Nonalcoholic beverages may be fine, but even some de-alcoholized drinks contain small amounts of the drug.

ALCOHOL DETOXIFICATION

Diet and megavitamin therapy are helpful during withdrawal, detoxification, and recovery. Certainly, people who use alcohol excessively need more supplements than others, and during detox they may require even more. During the actual withdrawal period, diet should focus on fluids and alkaline foods. The appetite is usually not very strong at this time; liquids are easy to consume and will also help clear alcohol from the body. Water, diluted fruit and vegetable juices, warm broths, soups, and teas using herbs such as chamomile, skullcap (a nervine), or valerian root are good choices. Other helpful herbs include white willow bark for reducing pain and inflammation, ginseng,

cayenne, and peppermint. Small amounts of light proteins, such as nonfatty poultry, fish, or even chicken soup will provide more nourishment. Amino acid powder is also supportive. L-glutamine, an amino acid, has been shown to reduce cravings for alcohol and sugar, and is used in many detox clinics. L-tryptophan and 5-HTP (5-hydroxy-tryptophan) support serotonin, which helps calm the nervous system and support sleep, and can be taken at night as well as in the morning.

I have seen intravenous supplements work quite well during the withdrawal period, as well as during drinking times and afterward. Extra vitamin C, B-complex, and minerals such as calcium, magnesium, and potassium can be used intravenously, especially if supplements taken by mouth are not well tolerated. Vitamin C powder buffered with these minerals and mixed into water or juice is helpful during withdrawal and later during the detox period.

Alcohol detoxification continues for several weeks after withdrawal. During this recovery time, the body will eliminate alcohol and other toxins, and begin breaking down some of the stored fat. Balanced nourishment with a low-fat, moderate-protein, complex-carbohydrate diet is recommended. Because alcoholics often have blood sugar problems, basic hypoglycemic principles should also be followed. These include avoiding sugars and refined foods such as soft drinks or candy, and eating every few hours. The basic diet consists of small meals and snacks of protein or complex carbohydrates, including whole grains like brown rice, pasta, potatoes, squashes, legumes, and other vegetables. Proteins such as soy products, sprouted beans, some nuts and seeds, eggs, fish, and poultry can also be added, and some fruits and fruit juices may be tolerated well. Because the primary aim is to maintain an alkaline diet, we should initially focus on vegetables and fruit. Of course, the Detox Diet can be used during the first two weeks of alcohol detoxification.

Water or herbal teas should be consumed throughout the day. Foods containing potentially damaging fats such as fast foods, lunch meats, chips, burgers, hot dogs, and ice cream should also be avoided, as they are all congesting and more acid-forming. Caffeine consumption and cigarette smoking are best minimized. Many people recovering from alcohol addiction consume large amounts of coffee and smoke intensely—an event seen clearly at some AA meetings. I do not recommend this at all. Fortunately, there has been an increase in the number of nonsmoking AA meetings and in general, many people are aware of improving all health habits during recovery.

During detoxification from alcohol, as with the other substances, supplemental nutrients are helpful. Herbal formulas, such as valerian root capsules, or prescription medicines can be used for sleep, as can 500 to 1,000 mg of L-tryptophan or 100 to 200 mg of 5-HTP. Calcium and magnesium supplements taken at night may also aid sleep. L-glutamine, an amino acid that generates glutamic acid, can be used

for energy. Glutamine is found naturally in liver, meats, dairy foods, and cabbage, and helps diminish the craving for alcohol and sugar. A supplement amount of 500 to 1,000 mg three times daily between or before meals is suggested, either in capsule or in powdered form. Chromium may also help with sugar and alcohol cravings; take 200 mcg twice daily. Melatonin can also be used and has had some good effects during detox for aiding sleep. One 3-mg tablet (the sublingual variety is best) can be taken at bedtime. There are also time-released tablets.

A multiple vitamin with additional antioxidant nutrients is a good idea during detox from alcohol. Minerals such as zinc, iron, calcium, and magnesium should be taken to replace those lost during alcohol abuse. Higher levels of niacin, even up to 2 grams, along with 5 to 10 grams of vitamin C daily, have been used with some success during alcohol withdrawal and detox. For basic support, vitamin C intake would be 500 to 1,000 mg taken four to six times daily.

Fiber helps bind toxins in the bowel and improves elimination. Choline and inositol, in doses of about 500 mg each three times daily, will improve fat digestion and utilization. Lemon water combined with a couple of teaspoons of olive oil and ¼ teaspoon or capsule of cayenne pepper will help detoxify the liver. You can decrease the oil absorption by taking fiber along with it, but olive oil alone is also thought to be nourishing to the liver and helpful in clearing chemical toxins. Cold-pressed olive oil is commonly used in many natural liver therapies. Milk thistle herb (*Silybum marianum* or silymarin) offers protection and healing to the liver during detoxification; taking between 60 and 100 mg twice daily is suggested. Taking one or two capsules of goldenseal root powder twice daily for a week or two is also helpful for toning and cleaning the liver. Parsley tea improves kidney elimination and cleanses the blood. The amino acid L-cysteine is another helpful detoxifier for the liver, blood, and colon.

Other nutrients and herbs can also be helpful. These include pancreatic digestive enzymes, taken after meals, and Brewer's yeast if tolerated, which supplies many B vitamins and minerals. The essential fatty acids help decrease the inflammatory prostaglandins. Gamma-linolenic acid from evening primrose or borage seed oil assists in the reduction of alcohol toxicity. White willow bark tablets can be used for pain, and valerian root, a natural and milder form of Valium, can be taken to decrease anxiety. Chamomile will help calm the digestive tract, as will licorice root.

NUTRITIONAL SUPPORT FOR DRINKERS

The basic support plan for active drinkers resembles that which is used during complete alcohol detoxification. A generally balanced and nutritious diet will help minimize some of the potential problems from alcohol, although even the best diet and supplement program will not fully protect us from ethanol's toxic effects. When our liver is metabolizing alcohol, it is helpful to avoid fried foods, rancid or hydrogenated fats, and other drugs, all of which are hard on the liver. Alpha-lipoic (thioctic) acid may help protect the liver against some of the toxicity, as can milk thistle herb. R-lipoic acid is also available and may be even more effective.

Alcohol users need more nutrients than most people to protect them from malnutrition. Obviously, basic multivitamins and antioxidant formulas are important. Part, or possibly most, of the toxic effects of alcohol may be caused by the production of free radicals. Higher-than-DRI (Daily Recommended Index) levels of vitamins A, C, and E, mixed carotenes, and the minerals selenium, zinc, manganese, and magnesium are suggested (for all dosages, see page 182). Commonly deficient nutrients also need extra support. Thiamine, riboflavin, and niacin help circulation and blood cleansing and can reduce the effects of hangovers. I recommend folic acid in an amount more than twice the DRI be taken; leafy greens and whole grains, both rich in this vitamin, should be added to the diet.

Water and other nonalcoholic liquids are needed to counteract the dehydrating effects of alcohol. Calcium is supportive, as is extra zinc, because its absorption is diminished and elimination is increased with alcohol use. This supplemental intake should be balanced out with copper. The essential fatty acids and gamma-linolenic acid from evening primrose oil or borage seed oil support normal fat metabolism and protect against inflammation caused by free radicals and prostaglandins (PGEs). Alcohol decreases the levels of the anti-inflammatory PGE1, and these oils will begin to raise their levels again. Glutathione helps prevent fat buildup in the liver through its enzymatic activities, so the tripeptide glutathione (or L-cysteine, which forms glutathione in the body) may be supplemented along with basic L-amino acids. Additional L-glutamine will enhance brain cell function.

SOCIAL DRINKING

I recommend that social drinkers use a lighter version of this program, because they still need protection against alcohol's toxicity. A good diet is, of course, essential, plus vitamins B_1, B_2, and B_3, folic acid, and B_{12}. These, along with zinc (15 to 30 mg), magnesium (300 to 500 mg), and vitamin C (1,000 mg), should be taken with some food before drinking. In general, drinking should be limited to two drinks per day.

A number of things can help prevent drunkenness and hangover. Our alcohol blood level is affected by how much and how fast we drink and absorb. Drink slowly. If we drink fast on an empty stomach, absorption is immediate. Ideally, it is best to have some food in the stomach or to limit consumption to one drink before eating. Food also prevents us from getting sick. We recommend low-salt complex carbohydrates such as whole-grain bread,

crackers, or vegetable sticks, because carbohydrates delay alcohol absorption. Fat-protein snacks such as milk, cheese, or nuts and seeds (such as almonds and sunflower seeds) will also decrease alcohol absorption, thus reducing drunkenness and hangovers. Some people even drink a little olive oil before parties to coat their stomachs before drinking. A few capsules of evening primrose oil will have a similar effect. Women seem to be more readily affected by alcohol than men, even when body weight is equal.

Once alcohol is ingested, it just takes time to clear it from the blood. With heavy drinking, extra coffee and exercise do not really help; however, with mild intoxication they can increase alertness. Definitely avoid other psychoactive drugs when drinking alcohol, including tranquilizers, narcotics, sedatives, antihistamines, and marijuana, all of which may increase alcohol's effect.

Alcohol blood levels have been studied in order to understand their varying effect. Tests are used to clarify degrees of safety while under the influence, versus more potentially dangerous drunkenness. Usually one or two drinks will leave people in the safe range, but more can create problems. Hangovers are caused both by the dehydrating effect of alcohol and by the toxic effects of the chemical congeners or sulfur compounds created during fermentation or added to the beverages. Allergies to some of the ingredients such as corn, wheat, barley, or yeast may intensify hangovers and withdrawal.

Blood Alcohol Content (BAC)	Status and Typical Experience[19]
0.06% BAC (Blood Alcohol Content)	Peak stimulation; after this, fewer positive effects. All emotions intensified.
0.07 to 0.09% BAC	Slight impairment of balance, speech, vision, reaction time, and hearing; still euphoric, yet judgment and self-control are reduced, with caution, reason, and memory being impaired.
0.08% BAC	Legally impaired. It is illegal to drive at this level. You will probably believe that you are functioning better than you really are.
0.10 to 0.15% BAC	Significant impairment of motor coordination and loss of good judgment. Speech may be slurred; balance, vision, reaction time, and hearing will be impaired. Euphoria often changes to anxiety.
0.16 to 0.19% BAC	Dysphoria predominates and nausea may appear. The drinker has the appearance of a "sloppy drunk."
0.20% BAC	Feeling dazed, confused, or otherwise disoriented. May need help to stand or walk. Some people experience nausea and vomiting. The gag reflex is impaired and you can choke if you do vomit. Blackouts are likely at this level, so you may not remember what has happened.
0.25% BAC	All mental, physical, and sensory functions are severely impaired. Increased risk of asphyxiation from choking on vomit and of seriously injuring yourself by falls.
0.3% BAC	Stupor. Little comprehension of where you are. You may pass out suddenly and be difficult to awaken.
0.35% BAC	Coma is possible. This is the level of surgical anesthesia.
0.40% BAC and above	Onset of coma, and possible death due to respiratory arrest.

Note: When BAC slowly rises and remains under 0.06%, the drinker is in the "buzz" or "cruising" zone. At this point, the drinker is feeling good, euphoric, and more sociable, with increased energy.

Blood alcohol content (BAC) refers to the amount of alcohol in milligrams per 100 milliliters of blood, usually expressed as a percentage. A BAC of 0.1 percent is equivalent to one part alcohol for every 1,000 parts of blood. Because drawing blood is not always practical, the easiest way to estimate BAC is by using a breathalyzer test that takes a sample of alveolar (deep lung) air.[20]

HANGOVER REMEDIES

The best hangover remedy is to not overdrink and to take supportive fluids and nutrients. Cream, coffee, oysters, chili peppers, and aspirin are common and occasionally helpful remedies. Time is the only real remedy, however, along with rest and fluids. If alcohol intake has been excessive, drink two or three glasses of water before going to bed, along with some vitamin C and a B-complex vitamin to clear alcohol from the blood. Repeat upon waking. Emergen-C or Power Pak can also be used—they are vitamin C powders with added vitamins and minerals, and are available at natural food stores. Evening primrose oil and flaxseed oil also help. A morning-after plan suggested by Dr. Stuart Berger includes 100 mg of thiamine, 100 mg of riboflavin, 50 mg of B_6, 250 mcg of B_{12} (a good B-complex can be used for these four vitamins, plus others), 1,000 mg of vitamin C, and 50 mg of zinc.

Overall, we need to monitor our drinking and not let alcohol use turn into abuse and addiction. We also need to pay special attention to children and teenagers and offer them education regarding alcohol and drugs and provide them with good role models in ourselves. Let us all live as examples of how we would like the world to be.

ALCOHOL NUTRIENT PROGRAMS

	Support	Withdrawal	Detox/Recovery
Water	2$\frac{1}{2}$ to 3 qt	3 to 4 qt	3 qt
Protein	60 to 80 g	50 to 70 g	75 to 100 g
Fats and oils	30 to 50 g	30 to 50 g	50 to 65 g
Fiber	15 to 20 g	10 to 15 g	30 to 40 g
Vitamin A	5,000 to 10,000 IU	5,000 IU	5,000 to 10,000 IU
Mixed carotenes	25,000 IU	20,000 IU	20,000 IU
Vitamin D	1,000 to 2,000 IU	1,000 to 2,000 IU	1,000 to 2,000 IU
Vitamin E	400 to 800 IU	400 IU	800 IU
Vitamin K	300 mcg	300 mcg	500 mcg
Thiamine (B$_1$)	100 mg	50 to 100 mg	150 mg
Riboflavin (B$_2$)	100 mg	50 to 100 mg	150 mg
Niacinamide (B$_3$)	50 mg	50 mg	50 mg
Niacin (B$_3$)	50 to 150 mg	100 to 1,000 mg	200 to 2,000 mg
Pantothenic acid (B$_5$)	250 mg	1,000 mg	500 mg
Pyridoxine (B$_6$)	100 mg	200 mg	100 mg
Pyridoxal-5-phosphate	50 mg	100 mg	50 mg
Cobalamin (B$_{12}$)	100 mcg	200 mcg	250 mcg
Folic acid	800 to 1,000 mcg	1,000 to 2,000 mcg	800 mcg
Biotin	300 mcg	500 mcg	500 mcg
Choline	500 mg	1,000 mg	1,500 mg
Inositol	500 mg	1,000 mg	1,500 mg
Vitamin C	2 to 4 g	5 to 25 g	5 to 10 g
Bioflavonoids	250 mg	500 mg	500 mg
Calcium*	600 to 1,000 mg	1,000 to 1,500 mg	1,000 mg
Chromium	500 mcg	500 to 1,000 mcg	300 mcg
Copper*	3 mg	3 mg	3 to 4 mg

	Support	Withdrawal	Detox/Recovery
Iodine	150 mcg	150 mcg	150 mcg
Iron*	10 to 30 mg	10 to 18 mg	10 to 20 mg
Magnesium*	500 to 800 mg	800 to 1,000 mg	600 to 800 mg
Manganese	5 mg	15 mg	10 mg
Molybdenum	300 mcg	300 mcg	300 mcg
Potassium*	300 to 500 mg	500 mg	300 mg
Selenium	300 mcg	150 mcg	200 mcg
Silicon	100 mg	50 mg	200 mg
Vanadium	150 mcg	150 mcg	150 mcg
Zinc*	45 to 75 mg	50 to 75 mg	50 to 100 mg
Flaxseed oil or	1 teaspoon	2 teaspoons	2 teaspoons
Omega-3 oils	2 to 4 capsules	3 to 6 capsules	2 to 4 capsules
Gamma-linolenic acid (40 to 60 mg/ capsule)	3 capsules	3 capsules	6 capsules
L-amino acids	1,000 to 1,500 mg	1,500 to 3,000 mg	5,000 to 7,500 mg
L-glutamine	500 to 1,000 mg	1,500 to 3,000 mg	1,000 to 2,000 mg
Lipoic acid	100 mg	100 mg	200 mg
L-cysteine or	250 mg	250 mg	250 to 500 mg
Glutathione	250 mg	500 mg	250 mg
Digestive enzymes	—	—	1 to 2 after meals
Goldenseal root	—	—	3 capsules
White willow bark (for pain)	1 to 2 tablets	4 to 6 tablets	2 to 4 tablets
Silymarin (milk thistle) (60 to 80 mg/cap or tab)	2 to 4 capsules	3 capsules	3 to 6 capsules

* Amounts may vary based on gender and individual needs.

ALCOHOL DETOX SUMMARY

1. If you have been **drinking for a long time or drink large amounts,** seek multileveled support. This gives you the best chance for a permanent change. Also, have some professional support and guidance for this detox process.

2. If you consume **more than six to eight drinks daily,** seriously consider inpatient help or a residential detox program. Most are thirty days or longer because it takes some work both physically and psychologically to change habits.

3. The **Juice Cleanse** (page 73) or the **Detox Diet** (page 68), often accompanied with light protein and amino acids, can be useful in the transition and detox process. Post-detox, whole foods with complex carbohydrates and adequate proteins can be nourishing.

4. Follow basic **hypoglycemic guidelines**—avoid sugars and sweetened foods, have some nourishment regularly (every two to three hours), and maintain adequate protein intake.

5. **Drink 6 to 8 glasses or more of water** daily to help clear the liver and cleanse the body of toxins.

6. **Include sufficient fiber** to support proper bowel elimination.

7. **Use nutritional supplements** to support your body during detoxification from alcohol. Medically supervised intravenous (IV) nutrition of vitamins B and C along with minerals may also be useful.

8. Be sure to include **antioxidant nutrients** to help with detox—namely, vitamins C and E, beta-carotene, zinc, and selenium.

9. Use **specific herbs** to cleanse and heal the liver and facilitate detoxification—these include milk thistle (silymarin), dandelion root, and others.

10. **Consider acupuncture** to treat physical cravings and withdrawal symptoms.

11. **Get support that fits** your own values—perhaps psychological counseling, family therapy, AA, or a religious or spiritual practice.

12. **Avoid places** and people that most trigger your drinking.

13. **Evaluate yourself**—when and how were you first introduced to drinking? When did it become a problem both emotionally and physically? Keep a journal so you can track your personal process.

Endnotes

1. Dietary guidelines for Americans 2010, US Depts of Agriculture and Health and Human Services.www.dietary guidelines.gov.

2. Sondra Barrett, *Wine's Hidden Beauty*, Mystic Molecules Media (2009): 64–66.

3. Earl S. Ford, MD, et al., "Low-Risk Lifestyle Behaviors and All-Cause Mortality: Findings from the National Health and Nutrition Examination Survey III Mortality Study," *American Journal of Public Health* 101, no. 10 (October 2011): 1922–9.

4. www2.potsdam.edu/hansondj/AlcoholAnd Health.html.

5. www.cdc.gov/alcohol/fact-sheets/alcohol-use. htm; D.A. Dawson, B.F. Grant, "Quantifying the Risks Associated with Exceeding Recommended Drinking Limits," *Alcohol Clinical and Experimental Research* 29 (2005): 902–8.

6. www.gallup.com/poll/141656/drinking-rate-edges-slightly-year-high.aspx.

7. www.cdc.gov/alcohol.

8. S. Nolen-Hoeksema, "Gender Differences in Risk Factors and Consequences for Alcohol Use and Problems," *Clinical Psychology Review* 24 (2004): 981.

9. http://promises.com/promisesnews/articles/ alcoholabuse/problem-drinking-a-greater-threat-than-recognized.

10. www.cdc.gov/alcohol/fact-sheets/underage-drinking.htm.

11. Office of Applied Studies, *Results from the 2008 National Survey on Drug Use and Health: National Findings* (Rockville, MD: Substance Abuse and Mental Health Services Administration, 2009). Available at http://www.samhsa.gov/data/ nsduh/2k8nsduh/2k8Results.pdf. (Accessed November 26, 2011).

12. R.W. Hingson, T. Heeren, and M.R. Winter, "Age at Drinking Onset and Alcohol Dependence: Age at Onset, Duration, and Severity," *Pediatrics* 160 (2006): 739–46; Office of Applied Studies, *Alcohol Dependence or Abuse and Age at First Use* (Rockville, MD: Substance Abuse and Mental Health Services Administration, 2004). Available at www.oas.samhsa.gov/2k4 /ageDependence/ageDependence.htm. (Accessed March 31, 2008.)

13. D.A. Dawson, B.F. Grant, F.S. Stinson, P.S. Chou, B. Huang, and W. Ruan, "Recovery from DSM-IV Alcohol Dependence: United States, 2001–2002," *Addiction* 100, no. 3 (2005): 281–92.

14. 2010 Status Report on United States' and Missouri's Alcohol and Drug Abuse Problems.

15. The Treatment Episode Data Set (TEDS) part of The National Survey of Substance Abuse Treatment Services (N-SSATS), Office of Applied Studies, Substance Abuse and Mental Health Services Administration (SAMHSA).

16. See note 13 above.

17. www.caron.org/current-statistics.html.

18. C. M. Chen and H. Yi, *Trends in Alcohol-Related Morbidity Among Short-Stay Community Hospital Discharges, United States, 1979–2005* (Bethesda, MD: National Institutes of Health, National Institute on Alcohol Abuse and Alcoholism, NIAAA Surveillance Report #80, 2007).

19. www.brad21.org/effects_at_specific_bac.html.

20. www.rochester.edu/uhs/healthtopics/Alcohol/ bac.html.

CHAPTER THIRTEEN
Caffeine Detoxification

CAFFEINE IS A WORLDWIDE UBIQUITOUS DRUG. Coffee, brewed from the ground coffee bean (*Coffea arabica*), is the major vehicle for caffeine consumption. Used originally in most cultures for ceremonies, it has become an overused energy stimulant in the Western world, with the United States leading in coffee and caffeine use. In 2010, the global consumption of coffee was 14 billion pounds, with Americans consuming 400 million cups per day, or 146 billion cups per year, making us the world's largest consumer of coffee.[1] Japan ranks third in the world for coffee consumption after the United States and Europe.[2]

In this country, more than half the people over age eighteen drink coffee, with most of them consuming three or more cups a day.[3] This food/drug mixture—often combined with sugar and/or milk—is one of the most highly marketed, addictive substances in the world. In fact, coffee trends in the United States are toward drinking more specialty coffees (such as espresso, cappuccino, and lattes).[4] And with the expansion of Starbucks, there are literally coffee shops on most corners in big cities and readily accessible throughout most Westernized countries. Let's face it: it's very easy to get caffeine everywhere, including coffee and colas at many types of stores.

There are several basic areas of concern with coffee consumption beyond caffeine intake, not the least of which focuses on the toxic chemicals used in growing and processing coffee. The oils in the beans easily go rancid and the irritating acids in beans offer further hazards. And, while over the last few decades there has been an increase in organically grown coffee, there has also been an increase in the use of pesticides and chemical processing. People trying to cut down on caffeine by drinking decaffeinated coffee could be exposed to other dangerous chemicals unless they are drinking water-processed decaf and using organically grown beans. This Swiss process uses steam distillation to remove the caffeine, whereas regular decaffeination uses agents such as trichlorethylene (TCE) and methylene chloride, which leave residues in the prepared decaf coffee itself.

Cocoa beans, used in making hot chocolate, also contain caffeine. In general, tea contains much less caffeine than coffee—where an average 8-ounce cup of coffee contains about 130 mg, the same size cup of black tea has 53 mg.[5] But all black or common teas such as Earl Grey or English Breakfast contain not only caffeine but also theophylline and theobromine, as do many green teas, with similar stimulating effects. Tannic acid, a mild irritant to the gastrointestinal mucosa that may reduce absorption of minerals such as manganese, zinc, and copper, can be found in both coffee and tea. Most herbal teas do not contain caffeine, although maté and guarana are fairly high in caffeine. Ephedra or mahuang is a Chinese herb that provides caffeine-like stimulation. These natural products have been used as stimulants throughout history. There is recent concern with ephedra (and guarana less so) products that are used for energy and weight loss, and they are now much less available due to FDA regulations. Many people have problems with nervousness, agitation, fast heart rate, palpitations, and even more dangerous heart issues. There have been some deaths from ephedra use/

overuse, and because of this, government legislation has helped eliminate ephedra stimulants from the public marketplace.

Another issue with caffeine is its widespread use as an added ingredient in products, including some soft drinks, energy bars, and many over-the-counter drugs. Some common pharmaceutical preparations contain caffeine for its stimulating effects, which counteract the sedating antihistamines, or for its cerebral vasodilating effects used to relieve vascular headaches. Cafergot is a prescription drug containing caffeine and is used for migraines; although caffeine can help reduce headaches, it more commonly causes them.

The problem here is less with caffeine as a drug itself and more with the amounts consumed and the constant stimulation on which people come to depend many times daily, sometimes unknowingly. One big area of concern here is with children and teenagers, who may consume large amounts of caffeine when drinking soft drinks. Cola naturally contains caffeine, yet many soft drinks have additional amounts that promote an addiction to the drink. The new energy drinks (Red Bull, Rockstar, Amp, Full Throttle) create even more of a problem for individuals because of their very high caffeine content.[6] Energy drinks are beverages that contain caffeine, taurine, herbs, vitamins, and sugar or corn sweeteners and are the fastest growing beverage market in the United States. Sales are expected to top $9 billion in 2011. These drinks have been associated with increased seizures, stroke, and sudden death.[7] Cocoa, which also contains caffeine, is also a popular beverage with kids in the United States.

Caffeine is often consumed along with other substances such as nicotine and sugar. In fact, some of the latest energy drinks also contain alcohol. Like sugar, caffeine overstimulates the adrenals and then weakens them with persistent or chronic use. A cycle develops where first sugar stimulates and weakens the adrenals, creating fatigue, to which we then respond by drinking caffeine to stay awake. In addition, people who overuse caffeine tend to need more tranquilizers and sleeping pills to help them relax or sleep because their nervous system remains overstimulated. Caffeine is often a lifetime drug for many. We begin at a young age with hot chocolate or chocolate bars, move into colas or other soft drinks, and then add coffee and tea. Of course, like any substance, when it's used on occasion, we can experience the benefits with less negative effects.

Physiologically, caffeine is a central nervous system (CNS) stimulant. It is a member of the class of methylxanthine chemicals/drugs. Xanthines (specifically theophylline) are commonly used in medicine to aid in breathing. Theobromine, another xanthine derivative, is found in cocoa. Methylxanthines are found in many other plants, including the kola nut originally used to make cola drinks.

A dosage of 50 to 100 mg of caffeine, the amount in one standard (6-ounce) cup of coffee, will produce a temporary increase in mental clarity and energy levels while simultaneously reducing drowsiness. It also improves memory and muscular-coordinated work activity, such as typing. Through its CNS stimulation, caffeine increases brain activity; however, it also stimulates the cardiovascular system, raising blood pressure and heart rate. It generally speeds up our body by increasing our basal metabolic rate which burns more calories. Initially, caffeine may lower blood sugar; however, this can lead to increased

---

CAFFEINE WITHDRAWAL SYMPTOMS

Headache	Craving	Irritability
Insomnia	Fatigue	Depression
Apathy	Constipation	Anxiety
Nervousness	Shakiness	Dizziness
Drowsiness	Inability to concentrate	Runny nose
Nausea	Vomiting	Cramps
Ringing in the ears	Feeling hot and cold	Tachycardia

hunger or cravings for sweets. After adrenal stimulation, blood sugar rises again. Caffeine also increases respiratory rates, and for people with tight airways, it can open breathing passages (as do the other xanthine drugs). Caffeine is also a diuretic and a mild laxative.[8]

The amount of caffeine needed to produce stimulation increases with regular use, as is typical of all addictive drugs. Larger and more frequent doses are needed to achieve the original effect, and symptoms can develop if we do not get our "fix." Eventually, we need the drug to function; without it, fatigue, drowsiness, and headaches can occur.

Unfortunately, most caffeine products do not contain any of the nutrients, such as manganese and copper, needed to support the increased activity that they cause. Also, the diuretic effect of caffeine leads to

the urinary loss of many nutrients, which frequently go unreplaced.

Overall, addiction to caffeine is not as bad as addiction to most other drugs. Usually, the slower the tapering of use, the easier the withdrawal. After complete withdrawal and detoxification from caffeine, it is possible to use it in moderation, but care must be taken because it can be readdicting.

The most common caffeine withdrawal symptom is a throbbing and/or pressure headache, usually located at the temples but occasionally at the back of the head or around the eyes. A vague muscular headache often follows. Of course, caffeine can cure these symptoms, but this is not the answer. Rather, we need to adhere to dietary guidelines and supplements to help with this and other withdrawal problems. It is best to taper off caffeine before going on a cleanse because the withdrawal (mainly headaches) can be very uncomfortable. The Detox Diet works well for this transition.

Fortunately, two noncaffeine trends related to beverage intake are evident: people are developing healthier habits by drinking more light fruit juices, fresh vegetables juices, and water. From 1980 to 1993, the average intake of bottled water increased from 2.4 to 9.2 gallons. Then, by 2005, Americans drank 25 gallons of bottled water per capita.[9] In 2008 alone, U.S. bottled water sales topped 8.6 billion gallons for 28.9 percent of the U.S. liquid beverage market. And, in 2010, the

---

CAFFEINE DRUGS AVAILABLE OVER THE COUNTER

Stimulants: No-Doz, Vivarin (1 tab 100 mg)

Weight control: Dexatrim Max Complex 7

Pain relief: Excedrin Extra Strength (2 tabs 130 mg), Anacin Maximum Strength (2 tabs 64 mg), and Vanquish

Menstrual pain relief: Midol Complete

Cold remedies: Dristan

world bottled water market represented an annual volume of 50 billion gallons.

Caffeine, although it is not seriously addicting, is very habit forming. I suggest that anyone interested in high-level health should avoid it. Although it may improve short-term performance, it eventually creates long-term depletion.

NEGATIVE EFFECTS OF CAFFEINE

Most of the negative effects of caffeine are not a concern with occasional use, but can occur with regular use of more than 100 mg daily. The risks vary with the level of caffeine intake and individual sensitivity. A total of more than 500 mg of caffeine daily is a high intake, and the total encompasses all sources, including coffee, tea, soft drinks, and drugs. (Remember that an average 6-ounce cup of coffee contains 130 mg of caffeine, black tea has 53 mg.) Between 250 and 500 mg can be classified as moderate intake, while less than 250 mg daily would be low. For a long time, the popularity of caffeine outweighed its negative effects. Although there are dangers, there is great controversy over the health risks and benefits of coffee consumption.[10] The benefits have been attributed to its many phytochemical and antioxidant components. Numerous research investigations have demonstrated that coffee consumption may lower the risk of type 2 diabetes, various cancers, Parkinson's disease, and Alzheimer's disease and improves cognitive function.[11] In its May 2011 issue, *The Journal of the National Cancer Institute* published the results of a study of almost 50,000 men that found heavy coffee drinkers (six cups a day) were less likely to develop prostate cancer over two decades than men who drank none.[12]

On the other hand, caffeine can raise serum cholesterol, posing a possible threat to coronary health and cardiovascular complications. Caffeine consumption contributes to insomnia, and its withdrawal is

---

SIGNS AND SYMPTOMS OF CAFFEINE INTOXICATION OR ABUSE

Nervousness	Anxiety	Irritability
Agitation	Tremors	Insomnia
Depression	Headache	Upset stomach
Gastrointestinal irritation	Heartburn	Diarrhea
Fatigue	Dizziness	Increased heart rate
Irregular heartbeat	Elevated blood pressure	Increased cholesterol
Nutritional deficiencies	Poor concentration	Bed wetting

accompanied by muscle fatigue and other problems in those addicted to coffee. Evidence shows that pregnant women or those with postmenopausal problems should avoid excessive consumption of coffee because it interferes with hormones.[13]

Although caffeine has the overall effect of increasing blood sugar, stress and sugar intake weaken adrenal function. Recovery from the resulting fatigue requires rest, stress reduction, and sugar avoidance, and even though caffeine can override this fatigue and restimulate the adrenals temporarily, eventually chronic fatigue, adrenal exhaustion, and subsequent inability to handle any stress or sugar will result. Caffeine will then be of little help.

DETOXIFICATION FROM CAFFEINE

People with a regular caffeine habit should seriously consider discontinuing its use until they can reach a state of occasional enjoyment. If addiction is clear, or if pregnant, caffeine should be given up completely. Breaking the habit by either tapering off or going cold turkey will be easier with a good diet and adrenal support. Also, anyone with a regular habit should take a one- or two-week break once or twice a year if for no other reason than to maintain a healthy relationship with coffee and its stimulating substance, caffeine. This is the real coffee break! Over time, the consistent caffeine stimulation can cause what we call adrenal burnout

CASE STUDY: J.K., AGE 30

I am addicted to my daily latte. I have used coffee to pick me up when I am depressed or tired. After drinking it for years, I noticed that I didn't get a rush from it anymore. In fact, it made me feel more tired.

Author's note: What J.K. is experiencing is adrenal depletion, which can happen from the overuse or abuse of stimulants. She quit coffee for three months and let her adrenal glands recover. Now she is out of the habit of using coffee and can safely enjoy an occasional cup without feeling drained. She said she also realizes now that she used to experience caffeine-induced anxiety. She is a much calmer and happier person now.

and an eventual fatigue/insomnia pattern with chronic stimulation that does not allow the proper recharging of the body's "batteries." This leads to a cycle of more and more coffee, trouble sleeping, more fatigue and coffee, and then increasing medical problems.

Two or three weeks of the Detox Diet can support the transition into a healthier and caffeine-free program. The post-detox diet includes vegetable salads, soups, greens, seaweed, some whole grains, various bean sprouts, and some nuts and seeds, using fruit for snacks. A decreased intake of acid foods such as meat, sugar, and refined flour products is also a good idea, as is avoiding the overuse of baked

CAFFEINE LEVELS* IN COMMON SUBSTANCES**

Coffee and Other Drinks (8 oz cup)	Amount of Caffeine (mg)
Drip	95 to 200
Instant	30 to 170
Decaf	2 to 12
Espresso (1 oz shot)	58 to 75
Caffe latte, Starbucks (16 oz)	150
Cappuccino	70
Caffe mocha	80
Brewed black tea (Earl Grey or English Breakfast)	40 to 120
Black tea, decaf	2 to 10
Green tea, Stash brand	30 to 40
Green Tea Drink, Arizona brand, 16 oz	15
Chocolate milk	10 to 15
Cocoa, Hershey's (dry, 1 tbsp)	40 to 50
Chocolate bar, Hershey's milk chocolate (1.55 oz)	9
Chocolate bar, Hershey's dark chocolate (1.45 oz)	31

* These caffeine levels and caffeine equivalents may depend on length of brewing time or amount of product used. The levels given are approximate.
** From the Center for Science in the Public Interest.

1) www.cspinet.org/new/cafchart.htm
2) www.mayoclinic.com/health/caffeine/AN01211
3) www.thehersheycompany.com/nutrition-and-wellness/chocolate-101/caffeine.aspx

goods (even whole-grain products), nuts, and seeds. Drinking at least 6 to 8 glasses of filtered water a day and sipping mineral water or herbal teas can help replace the coffee habit. Baking soda or, better, potassium bicarbonate tablets, will help make the body more alkaline and reduce some of the withdrawal symptoms.

In addition, vitamin C supplementation helps during withdrawal by supporting the adrenal glands. As a stress-reducer, several grams or more of vitamin C can be taken over the course of the day, preferably in a buffered form, especially with the main alkaline minerals—potassium, calcium, and magnesium—as well as zinc.

Soft Drinks (12 oz serving)	Amount of Caffeine (mg)
Colas	30 to 65 (colas are limited by the FDA to a maximum of 71 mg per serving)
Mountain Dew	54
Dr. Pepper, regular or diet	42 to 44
7-Up	0
Fanta, all flavors	0
Energy Drinks	
Red Bull, 8.3 oz	76
Rockstar, 8 oz	80
Monster Energy, 16 oz	160
OTC Medicines (all in mg/tablet)	
No-Doz	200
Vivarin	200
Dexatrim Max	200
Cafergot	100
Excedrin	65
Fiorinal	40
Anacin	30
Vanquish	35
Midol	30

I also suggest B-complex vitamins with extra pantothenic acid (250 mg four times daily), along with 500 mg of vitamin C every two or three hours.

During average coffee use, we need to be careful to replenish depleted nutrients, including thiamine (B_1), riboflavin (B_2), pyridoxine (B_6), vitamin C, potassium, magnesium, and, to a lesser degree, zinc, iron, calcium, and the trace minerals. Additional amino acids can help balance our energy level during use of or withdrawal from caffeine. Water intake and additional fiber will support bowel function, which frequently slows down during caffeine withdrawal.

COMMON NEGATIVE SIDE EFFECTS OF CAFFEINE

- Excess nervousness, irritability, insomnia, restless leg syndrome, dizziness, and subsequent fatigue

- Headaches

- Heartburn

- General anxiety (even panic attacks)

- Hyperactivity and bed wetting in children

- Increased stomach hydrochloric acid production (clearly problematic for people with existing ulcers or gastritis)

- Loss of minerals such as potassium, magnesium, and zinc, and vitamins including the B vitamins, particularly thiamine and vitamin C

- Reduced absorption of iron and calcium (especially when caffeine is consumed around mealtimes)

- Osteoporosis and anemia

- Interrupted growth in children and adolescents

- Diarrhea

- Increased blood pressure and hypertension, especially in atherosclerosis and heart disease

- Increased cholesterol and triglyceride blood levels

- Heart rhythm disturbances and mild arrhythmias, tachycardia, and palpitations

- Increased norepinephrine secretion, which causes some vasoconstriction (although caffeine may have mild vasodilating effects in the heart and body, excess adrenal stimulation may override this)

- Increase in cardiovascular disease risk factors, including homocysteine levels and blood pressure[14]

- Fibrocystic breast disease (again, results vary, but it is clear that some women experience an increase in size and number of cysts with increased use of caffeine)

- Kidney stones, which can occur as a result of the diuretic and chemical effects (adequate magnesium levels prevent calcification)

- Increased fevers, both as a direct effect and by counteracting the effect of aspirin

- Prostate enlargement may also be attributed to increased caffeine intake

- Adrenal exhaustion/stress/fatigue is tied to caffeine use

HERBAL CAFFEINE SUBSTITUTES

Roasted barley	Chicory root	Pero
Teechin	Postum	Rostaroma
Pioneer	Rombouts	Miso broth
Wilson's Heritage	Cafix	Ginseng root
Duran	Peppermint	Lemongrass
Gingerroot	Comfrey leaf	Red clover
Dandelion root		

GRAIN BEVERAGES FOR COFFEE SUBSTITUTES

Grain drink mixes are made of ingredients such as malt, chicory, barley, rye, figs, beet roots, and licorice. Brew according to directions on the package or as you would coffee. Add rice, hazelnut, or grain milks for a latte-like replacement drink.

Pioneer	Barley Coffee	Rombouts
Rostaroma	Inka	Raja's Cup
Cafix	Pero	Wilson's Heritage

Spreading the detoxification program over a week or two and reducing caffeine intake to none will help avoid significant headaches. Lower caffeine intake by drinking grain-coffee blends, diluted or smaller amounts of regular coffee, or decaffeinated coffee (water processed). Another approach is to first substitute black tea, which has less caffeine than coffee, and which can be tapered more easily.

If headaches occur, mild pain relievers can be used for a few days, but avoid taking them over a longer period of time. Increased water intake, vitamin C and mineral support, an alkaline diet, and white willow bark herb tablets, which contain a natural salicylate, should ease these withdrawal symptoms.

There are a number of herbal teas to use in place of coffee that can be both stimulating and refreshing. The roasted herbal roots, including barley, chicory, and dandelion, are most popular. Grain "coffees," such as Barley Coffee, Cafix, Inka, Pero, Rombouts, Raja's Cup, and Wilson's Heritage, are also favored among former coffee drinkers, while ginseng root tea is preferred by some. Teechino is a tasty and popular grain beverage that helps some coffee users transition to this healthier drink. Herbal teas made from lemongrass, peppermint, gingerroot, red clover, and comfrey are very nourishing, and do not have the depleting side effects. The algaes can also be energizing in place of caffeine.

If you do like to drink a cup of coffee or caffeinated tea a day, it might be best to drink it in the mid- to late afternoon, which is different from what most people do, using caffeine as their wake-up call and for energy through the day. The afternoon cup best fits our body's natural cycle, avoiding the high-adrenal morning and late pre-sleep hours. Those who cannot relax or sleep well after using caffeine should consider avoiding it altogether.

The pleasures of coffee and tea drinking are as much a cultural phenomenon as they are a taste preference. Remember, habits are developed, not inherent, and anything we learn, we can also unlearn or relearn.

Use the lower ranges of nutrients in the table opposite for general support and the higher levels for detoxification. The amounts shown are daily totals and should be divided into two or three supplementations during the day.

CAFFEINE DETOX SUMMARY

1. If you take in more than 500 mg a day of caffeine, consider taking a break from it, and clearing your body of caffeine. If you are pregnant and have a high caffeine intake, detox under the guidance of a health-care practitioner.

2. After that, avoid the daily use of caffeine. For most people, it can still be tolerated and enjoyed as long as it does not become a dependent daily habit.

3. Consider the Detox Diet or a general alkaline diet consisting mainly of vegetables, both steamed and as salads, fruits, some whole grains, and some protein, such as a few nuts or seeds, or a little fish or poultry if you feel it's needed.

4. Drink at least 6 to 8 glasses of water daily or more, especially if you exercise and sweat.

5. Keep fiber intake high to help clear the colon and support detoxification.

6. Supplement your nutrition with vitamins and minerals as outlined.

7. If headaches occur, as they commonly do in the first few days of detox, increase your intake of water, vitamin C, and minerals, and use white willow bark herb to ease headaches and withdrawal.

8. Other herbs, particularly as teas, can be taken to support the body or as coffee substitutes.

CAFFEINE SUPPORT AND DETOX NUTRIENT PROGRAM

Water	2½ to 3 qt		Bioflavonoids	250 to 500 mg
Fiber	15 to 20 g		Calcium	800 to 1,000 mg
Vitamin A	5,000 IU		Chromium	200 to 400 mcg
Mixed carotenoids	15,000 to 30,000 IU		Copper	2 to 3 mg
Vitamin D	400 to 2,000 IU		Iodine	150 mcg
Vitamin E	400 to 800 IU		Iron* (men)	0 to 15 mg
Vitamin K	300 mcg		Iron* (women)	15 to 30 mg
Thiamine (B₁)	75 to 150 mg		Magnesium	500 to 800 mg
Riboflavin (B₂)	50 to 100 mg		Manganese	5 to 10 mg
Niacinamide (B₃)	50 to 100 mg		Molybdenum	300 to 500 mcg
Niacin (B₃)	50 to 100 mg		Potassium	300 to 600 mg
Pantothenic acid (B₅)	500 to 1,000 mg		Silicon	50 to 100 mg
Pyridoxine (B₆) and/or	50 to 100 mg		Selenium	200 to 300 mcg
			Zinc	30 to 60 mg
Pyridoxal-5-phosphate	25 to 50 mg		Adrenal	50 to 150 mg
			L-amino acids	500 to 1,500 mg
Cobalamin (B₁₂)	100 to 200 mcg		Potassium bicarbonate**	600 to 1,000 mg
Folic acid	400 to 800 mcg			
Biotin	300 mcg		Herbal teas	3 cups daily
Vitamin C	2 to 6 g		Blue-green algae	500 to 2,000 mg

* Level would depend on lab values; otherwise, use only 10 mg/day maximum.
** Can use Alka-Seltzer Effervescent Antacid, one tablet two to three times daily. Antacids used excessively or with meals may interfere with proper digestion.

Endnotes

1. Isis Almeida, "Coffee Consumption Seen Rising in Emerging Market Countries," *Bloomberg*, September 14, 2011. www.bloomberg.com/news/2011-09-14/coffee-consumption-seen-rising-in-emerging-market-countries.html (accessed November 10, 2011).

2. Coffee-Statistics.com, "Coffee Statistics Report 2011 Edition." http://coffee-statistics.com/coffee_statistics_ebook.html (accessed November 10, 2011).

3. Harvard School of Public Health, "Coffee by the Numbers." www.hsph.harvard.edu/multimedia/flash/2010/coffee/facts.html (accessed November 10, 2011).

4. www.fao.org/fileadmin/templates/organic exports/docs/Market_Organic_FT_Coffee.pdf (accessed November 26, 2011).

5. Center for Science in the Public Interest, "Caffeine Content of Food and Drugs." www.cspinet.org/new/cafchart.htm (accessed November 26, 2011).

6. S.M. Seifert, J.L. Schaechter, E.R. Hershorin, and S.E. Lipshultz, "Health Effects of Energy Drinks on Children, Adolescents, and Young Adults," *Pediatrics* 127 (2011): 511–28.

7. Ibid.

8. J.V. Higdon and B. Frei, "Coffee and Health: A Review of Recent Human Research," *Critical Reviews of Food Science and Nutrition* 46, no. 2 (2006): 101–23.

9. "Changing Consumer Tastes Creates Explosive Growth for Domestic and International Bottled Water Brands—Revenue in 2007 Expected to Reach $5.974 Billion with Growth Set to Climb Higher Through 2012," press release, IBISWorld, May 21, 2008.

10. M.S. Butt and M.T. Sultan, "Coffee and Its Consumption: Benefits and Risks," *Critical Reviews in Food and Science Nutrition* 51, no. 4 (April 2011): 363–73.

11. K. Kempf et al., "Effects of Coffee Consumption on Subclinical Inflammation and Other Risk Factors for Type 2 Diabetes: A Clinical Trial," *American Journal of Clinical Nutrition* 91, no. 4 (April 2010): 950–7; See note 10 above.

12. K. M. Wilson et al., "Coffee Consumption and Prostate Cancer Risk and Progression in the Health Professionals Follow-up Study," *The Journal of the National Cancer Institute* 103, no. 19 (May 2011): 1481.

13. See note 10 above.

CHAPTER FOURTEEN

Chemical and Drug Detoxification

DRUG DETOXIFICATION INVOLVES two main processes—changing our abusive habits (not using the drugs) and releasing the drug residues from our bodies and our lives. This can be done even with decreased use of some drugs and medications.

We are a drug culture, and Western medicine is likewise a drug-oriented system. We consume billions of pills yearly and spend many billions of dollars buying them, as do our insurance companies and the government. These figures do not even begin to include the everyday use of caffeine, alcohol, and nicotine and how much money people spend on those products.

There are really no stereotypical drug addicts anymore. Affluent and poor people, and anyone under pressure or with unmet psychological needs, can end up with this problem. Substance abuse is an individual, family, and global problem that can affect young and old, men and women. And in truth, most people in modern Western cultures are addicted to one or more substances/drugs, sugar and caffeine being the most common.

It is important to understand the relationship between states of being, symptoms, and our use of drugs. When we choose to view a symptom as problematic, we want to correct it with drugs. Although for immediate relief this may seem practical, it is theoretically shortsighted and shows a complete misunderstanding of human body design. In actuality, drug use and drug therapy rarely fix anything. Our symptoms serve as a warning sign of some bigger problem for which we must determine the cause. Symptoms are not most often the real problem, but rather are the results of deeper processes and causes. They are also not errors on the part of our bodies, because the human body rarely errs; rather, our bodies respond to the way we treat them, just like any relationship. To correct aggravating symptoms, we must correct our internal imbalances and usually alter our lives. It is very important not to devitalize our body in any way if we can possibly avoid it. Because much habitual drug use is part of a syndrome of self-destruction, the first step for many people is to learn to care for and love themselves again, reinforcing their desire to live.

Pharmaceutical prescriptions and most over-the-counter (OTC) drugs are designed to help us feel better, yet they are too often used to treat problems resulting from abusive or misguided habits. This may aggravate the original problem or cause side effects. The promotion of addictions (which both support and drain our economy) begins with an emphasis on sugar. In fact, the use of sugar is so pervasive in our culture that it is difficult to find prepared or packaged foods that do not contain sugar or other sweeteners. Our habitual sweet tooth progresses to addictive usage of caffeine, nicotine, alcohol, and foods such as wheat, refined foods, and milk products. Later, the coffee break (combined with sugary snacks or coffee sweeteners) becomes a reward—a refueling rest stop during the workday. Caffeine and sugar stimulate us to work more. Nervousness and hyperactivity are often associated with productivity, although they are really not comparable to steady, healthful energy. Trying to perpetuate that productivity through the use of artificial stimulants eventually leads to reduced capacity, time lost from work, wasted money, and increased illness. Our behavior regarding foods, particularly sweet ones, is conditioned very early and is very difficult to change.

All drugs have some toxicity. Most have both physiological and psychological actions and addictive potential that result in accumulated toxicity and withdrawal symptoms when we try to give them up. **Before going through any drug or chemical detoxification, it is wise to prepare for the process.** This is important both physically and psychologically, and it is definitely helpful to have a physician or other health-care provider, therapist or counselor, family member or good friend for support. The withdrawal phase poses the most difficulties and can last from a day or two to a week or more. It is often hard to differentiate the physical sensations from the underlying psychological involvement. The withdrawal phase itself is part of the drug addiction cycle; in other words, the worse the withdrawal, the more likely we are to continue to use the chemical to prevent those symptoms. A psychological dependency easily develops from the physical dependency.

After the initial withdrawal, where we detoxify through the release of stored chemicals from the body, we need willpower and commitment to keep the particular substance out of our life. We also need to work on new behavior patterns, such as avoiding exposure to the people and places associated with our previous problem until we develop new habits. Those new habits need to be strong enough so that we can easily say no when we are exposed to the substance again. Behavior modification therapy can be very helpful.

Characteristics of addiction include needing the drug to function, needing it in ever higher doses, needing it more frequently, feeling sick when a dose is missed, and/or having a history of abuse or addiction. The most useful approach to dealing with drug addiction begins with admitting there is a problem. We must then combine our desire and willpower to accomplish this difficult task—detox and recovery—and there are many support programs and government resources to help. This decision often arises during illness or crisis rather than as a true desire to be healthy. Nonetheless, whatever gets us there is just fine, as long as we have the determination to follow through and stay on the path.

A well-balanced diet and a good nutritional supplement program are essential to an effective plan, as is some psychological support. During the transition, either a cleansing diet or a fast is helpful to enhance purification and lessen the severity and length of withdrawal. I have seen people make dramatic lifestyle changes with only a weeklong cleanse. Their new sense of empowerment helps them clarify their goals while reinforcing their willpower.

The Detox Diet program, which focuses primarily on steamed vegetables with some additional fruit and grains, allows a smooth transition with minimal withdrawal. It works to increase alkalinity and reduce acidity, which supports natural detoxification. Cravings and withdrawal intensify with an acid state generated by meats, milk products, and refined flours and sugars. A general diet that emphasizes fruits and vegetables, juices and soups, or even water can be used temporarily, as these are all alkaline-forming.

I do not suggest withdrawing or detoxifying from drugs during illness or either right before or after surgery, although sometimes it is unavoidable. However, during pregnancy (ideally before pregnancy), it is important to clear all unnecessary drugs, including OTC drugs, alcohol, nicotine, and caffeine. In all cases, we must be careful when withdrawing from these substances, although usually the basic daily habits can be tapered off and eliminated over the course of a few days. Because fetal stability is vitally important, it would be wise to have medical supervision during any form of detoxification during pregnancy.

Supplemental nutrients also support the system during drug elimination. Vitamin C and the other antioxidants—vitamins A and E, zinc and selenium, L-cysteine and other amino acids—are particularly important, in addition to a basic vitamin and mineral supplement. Glutathione, which is formed from L-cysteine in the body, acts with detoxification enzymes and helps decrease the toxicity of most drugs and chemicals.

A nutritional supplement approach to drug detoxification includes the B vitamins, minerals, a high amount of vitamin C, antioxidants, and the L-amino acids. These are more efficient when combined with a food diet than with fasting, and thus the alkaline, fruit- and vegetable-based diet is a better complement to any high nutrient intake. With a more liquid diet, minimize your intake of supplements and add more vitamin C, some minerals, and an antioxidant formula, along with herbs and chlorophyll or algae products.

Herbal therapies can also be helpful. Goldenseal root powder is probably the most important herb because it not only stimulates the liver to better perform its detoxifying function but also helps clear toxicity with its alkaloids. Take one large or two small capsules twice daily before meals for one or two weeks. Milk thistle, specifically *Silybum marianum*, also protects the liver from toxins and supports the detoxification process. Other helpful herbs during drug detoxification are those that work as laxatives, diuretics, and blood or lymph cleansers (see page 82 for a list of detoxifying herbs). Valerian root and other tranquilizing herbs may also lessen excitatory withdrawal symptoms such as anxiety or insomnia. Chlorophyll, taken as tablets or liquid, has a mildly purifying and rejuvenating quality.

PHARMACEUTICALS— PRESCRIPTION AND OTC DRUGS

Any prescription or OTC drug can be toxic, especially when used too much or for too long. Aspirin, anti-inflammatory and pain-relieving drugs, tranquilizers, and antidepressants are all in common use and are all similarly toxic, especially to the gastrointestinal tract and liver. The same is true for antibiotics, used millions of times a day across the country to treat many kinds of apparently infectious illnesses, which natural medicine thinkers believe are often the body's attempts to cleanse itself and heal by releasing mucus debris, creating fevers, and inflaming membranes. Regular use/overuse of these incredibly valuable treatments for bacterial infections also cause imbalances, allergic reactions, and digestive tract disturbances, altering normal flora (now referred to as *biome*). Keeping ourselves healthy and clear is the prime way to stay away from using these strong drug therapies.

In other words, the key to preventing the need to detoxify from drugs is to avoid their use in the first place. Many people are turning from Western medicine to alternative therapies and remedies (both traditional and modern) as better preparation and knowledge have improved their efficacy. When used correctly, they support the body's natural healing powers and correct imbalances. Consult with a knowledgeable practitioner or information source

COMMON OTC DRUGS

Symptoms commonly treated with OTC Drugs	Common OTC Drugs
Headache	Aspirin, acetaminophen, ibuprofen
Fatigue	Caffeine, nicotine, No-Doz
Insomnia	Tranquilizers
Colds, flu, and allergies	Antihistamines, decongestants
Constipation	Laxatives, lubricants
Diarrhea	Kaopectate, fibers
Indigestion	Antacids, Pepto-Bismol, Alka-Seltzer
Excess weight	Stimulants, such as ephedra and phentermine

for appropriate guidance, as herbs and other natural remedies (as well as homeopathy) can produce occasional side effects as well (or might interact with the other medicines you take). Acupuncture, osteopathic and chiropractic therapies, massage, and other bodywork can stimulate elimination and natural healing during detoxification periods.

Although OTC products are usually less toxic than pharmaceuticals, they are also more frequently abused because they can be readily obtained and are less expensive than most prescription drugs. Many symptoms are commonly treated with specific OTC drugs, as shown in the above chart.

Even at low potencies, many of these OTC drugs can create physical dependency. This is true especially when there is a chronic problem that requires long-term usage or when there are withdrawal or rebound symptoms. If problems persist, we should consult our health-care practitioner to help us determine the underlying cause and work to correct that rather than continue to treat the symptoms alone. If stress and worry are the cause of insomnia or if poor food choices or mealtimes lead to our gastrointestinal symptoms, we need to make some lifestyle changes. If the symptoms persist, herbs or homeopathy are typically more gentle remedies.

Aspirin and caffeine are at the top of the OTC drug problems list. (Caffeine is discussed thoroughly in chapter 13.) Aspirin, a valuable medicine in common use for many decades, is on the decline due to GI irritation and other concerns, although it is still used commonly in lower amounts for blood thinning in protecting against cardiovascular events. Acetaminophen (Tylenol), ibuprofen (Advil,

Motrin), and other anti-inflammatory medications (NSAIDs—non-steroidal anti-inflammatory drugs) have reduced the overall intake of aspirin. However, they come with their own health risks. Americans take on average twenty-four doses of NSAIDs per person per year, but because most don't take NSAIDs at all, the average dose is higher for those using these drugs. This class of medications irritates the intestinal lining, which leads to internal bleeding and ulcers in some cases. More than 100,000 people are hospitalized in the United States each year due to intestinal bleeding from NSAID use, accounting for $2 billion in health-care costs and 17,000 deaths.[1] Often those hospitalized use moderate doses. Many people use these medications at the first sign of swelling or discomfort, but they should only be used when necessary and after other more natural therapies are used. This includes massage, chiropractic, and Epsom salt baths for musculoskeletal pain; relaxation, rest, and detox for headaches; and herbal and nutritional products. Detox helps many aches and pains, so follow this book, and you won't need to call me in the morning.

Acetylsalicylic acid (the *aspirin* name is trademarked by Bayer), derived from coal tar, has more than 50 million regular users in this country consuming 20,000 tons of aspirin and 225 tablets per person per year in the United States. Globally, 80 billion aspirin tablets are taken each year.[2] Aspirin formulas often contain caffeine and act as anti-inflammatory agents. Aspirin works to reduce fevers (which, if left alone, are natural healers) and tends to work better than its counterpart acetaminophen. Both drugs are now in common use as people experience more pain and more degenerative conditions, such as arthritis and cardiovascular disease. Low doses of aspirin have been found to reduce blood-clotting effects and are commonly taken to reduce heart attack and stroke risk as one baby aspirin (81 mg) a day. (The typical aspirin tablet for adults is 325 mg, whereby two or three of those are taken to relieve the pain of arthritis, for example.)

The key to eliminating anti-inflammatory drugs is to eliminate the pain for which they are taken. Stronger pain medications include anti-inflammatories like ibuprofen and the relatively new Vioxx and Celebrex; most of these drugs have side effects, especially in the gastrointestinal tract. Vioxx was taken off the market for cardiovascular problems, and Celebrex, although helpful for arthritis, is still available but used less frequently due to similar concerns. Pain problems are frequently treated with even stronger prescription narcotics, such as codeine (aspirin or acetaminophen with codeine is very commonly used), hydrocodone (Vicodin), propoxyphene (Darvon), or even Demerol or morphine. All of these narcotic drugs are addictive and thus more difficult to stop using; however, they are tolerated better by some people than other medicines are.

TRANSITIONING FROM DRUGS TO NATURAL THERAPIES

I began studying and working with natural medicines only after I learned about and prescribed pharmaceutical drugs. Upon investigation, I became aware that many of the drugs I was prescribing had their basis or origin in plants. Some examples are Valium from valerian root, Ipecac from ipecaquana root, and Digoxin (digitalis) from the foxglove plant. Scientists studied the active plant ingredients and then synthesized like molecules and stronger variations of those phytochemicals.

Well, I think we lost something in the transition, namely, the safety and general positive effects of the plants with minimal side effects. We gained something also—power and speed and accurate dosages. These drugs have greater, though sometimes more limited, effects, and of course, they usually have side effects and potential toxicity.

Over the past three decades, I have taken a back-to-nature approach in my medical practice and my personal life. That means living more closely to and with greater reverence for nature, and thus paying closer attention to how I live. I eat more wholesomely and exercise and relax outdoors as often as possible. I have come to the awareness that my body is a part of nature, not separate from her. After more than thirty-five years of finely tuning this awareness, I have learned to sense more subtle adverse changes in my body. Because they are more subtle and less symptomatic, I can correct them with less invasive and safer therapies, specifically with dietary changes, nutritional supplements, herbal and homeopathic remedies, rest and quiet, and hands-on therapies like massage and chiropractic treatments.

I encourage you to try a natural remedy the next time you experience a problem, unless of course, you believe your condition to be serious or dangerous. Some common ailments with examples of natural therapies are in the box on page 205.

One of the most exciting and rewarding aspects of my "natural-first" medical practice is the positive results my patients experience with minimal or no side effects. In fact, they experience many **"side benefits" in feeling and looking better,** often with other symptoms getting better. Over the years, they've discovered for themselves that eating well and exercising regularly removes the need to even consider taking drugs because they don't get sick! Of course, if someone is acutely ill and/or in danger medically, I will use the quicker and stronger medications, and then later work to transition them to a more natural therapy. My philosophy of practice is simple—**lifestyle first, natural therapies next, and drugs last.**

Please realize that all treatments, be they dietary changes, nutritional supplements and herbs, or drugs, are an *experiment*, or more accurately, an *experience*. **Until you try any treatments yourself, you cannot really know their exact effect upon your symptoms, disease, or health.** To properly assess this personal experiment, be patient and be aware of and attentive to changes that occur. Initially, you may experience some adverse or unusual side effects, as in cleansing or healing reactions, but these should pass relatively quickly. (This is discussed more thoroughly in chapters 2 and 4.)

More commonly, and importantly, there are many positive side effects and healthful rewards to using natural therapies. Patients often report feeling clear-headed, physically energized, spiritually rejuvenated, and ready to set new goals and make new commitments. They look and feel younger, and have a vital, new sense of self with a more expansive and connected understanding. The key is to give nature a chance. After all, you didn't accumulate the excess weight, poor digestion, ill health, or addictive habits overnight.

OTHER DRUGS—STREET AND RECREATIONAL

Street or recreational **narcotics** are also a major social (and health) problem and generally pose a greater, though not insurmountable, challenge to detoxification.

These include opium, methadone, heroin, and crack. More than 3 million people over the age of twelve in the United States have tried heroin at least once.[3] It is estimated that there are between 750,000 and one million heroin addicts in the United States.[4] The drug creates a mix of euphoria and depression and also reduces the appetite and libido; in more extreme situations, basic life needs become less important than the user's focus on obtaining and ingesting the drug. There are many individuals who are in various stages of recovery from drugs, including alcohol and narcotics, and still others in methadone support centers. Dealing with drug dependence has many levels of cause and cure—physical, mental, emotional, and spiritual. Commitment to the path is a healthy philosophy in this regard.

In our medical system, there are many **prescription pill** habits begun and continued every year. Sleeping pills, tranquilizers, and antidepressants are all frequently prescribed and used to handle life's frustrations and challenges. In many instances, the problem is a poor diet and stress, and the daily use of stimulant and sedative substances (the SNACCs) as reviewed in this book; changing these lifestyle patterns may help alleviate the mood and energy dysfunctions that we just end up treating.

Valium was once the number one choice for stressed out and anxious people (starting with unhappy or frustrated housewives). Now, newer drugs such as Ativan, Xanax, and Buspar are gaining in popularity because they offer tranquilization and sedation to life's stresses. (Barbiturates used to be the main sedative but not now, although they are more frequently found as street drugs.) These drugs affect anxiety by depressing our nervous system in a way somewhat like alcohol. Use the principles and protocol described in the alcohol detoxification chapter (chapter 12) if these drugs are being taken.

Stimulants such as amphetamines and cocaine can cause dramatic fluctuations in energy. They excite the nervous system and promote euphoria or irritability but result in a loss of appetite, hypersensitivity, and insomnia, usually followed by fatigue and depression. The amphetamine stimulants like Dexedrine and Desoxyn, even though less popular than in prior years, still remain a problem for some. Nowadays, stimulants like Adderall and Concerta are used to treat ADHD (Attention Deficit Hyperactivity Disorder) in both children and adults. As with the narcotics, amphetamine withdrawal and detoxification from addiction often require professional assistance, although some people manage to do both on their own. The stimulant drugs, in general, are more deadly than others because they stress and damage the body (cocaine and amphetamines are known for this), so it is very important to eliminate them if we want to live long and healthfully.

Marijuana (*Cannabis sativa* and *C. indica*) has become the second most common drug used in the world after

DRUG DETOXIFICATION NUTRIENT PROGRAM

Water	2 to 3½ qt		Vitamin C	2 to 10 g
Fiber	20 to 40 g		Bioflavonoids	250 to 500 mg
Vitamin A	5,000 to 10,000 IU		Quercetin	250 to 600 mg
Mixed carotenoids	20,000 to 40,000 IU		Calcium	650 to 1,200 mg+
			Chromium	200 to 500 mcg
Vitamin D	400 to 2,000 IU		Copper	2 to 3 mg
Vitamin E	200 to 800 IU		Iodine	150 mcg
Vitamin K	300 mcg		Iron	10 to 20 mg**
Thiamine (B₁)	25 to 100 mg		Magnesium	400 to 800 mg+
Riboflavin (B₂)	25 to 100 mg		Manganese	5 to 10 mg
Niacinamide (B₃)	50 to 100 mg		Molybdenum	150 to 300 mcg
			Potassium	100 to 500 mg
Niacin (B₃)	50 to 1,000 mg*		Selenium	200 to 300 mcg
Pantothenic acid (B₅)	250 to 1,000 mg		Silicon	50 to 150 mg
			Vanadium	200 to 400 mcg
Pyridoxine (B₆) and/or	25 to 100 mg		Zinc	30 to 60 mg
Pyridoxal-5-phosphate	25 to 50 mg		L-amino acids	1,000 to 1,500 mg
			L-cysteine	250 to 500 mg
Cobalamin (B₁₂)	100 to 250 mcg		L-glutamine	250 to 1,000 mg
Folic acid	400 to 800 mcg		Essential fatty acids and/or	2 to 4 capsules
Biotin	300 mcg			
Choline	500 to 1,000 mg		Flaxseed oil	2 to 4 teaspoons
Inositol	500 to 1,000 mg		Goldenseal root	3 to 6 capsules

* Increase dosage slowly.
** As needed if low.

+ Higher amounts are needed for hyperactive withdrawal states, aches, or cravings.

alcohol (and not counting caffeine and sugar). And now with its medical effects and potential to help in some symptomatic situations (nausea, back pain, and headaches, as examples) as well as health conditions (pain from cancer and other diseases, and loss of appetite from AIDS), it has become a challenge to know how to proceed on a state and national level. Many states are seeking to legalize marijuana and at least decriminalize it. Hopefully, in the near future, it can be regulated like alcohol and nicotine and the governments can make the income needed to support the people rather than having this mostly tax-free (evaded) income go to the few growers and distributors.

Furthermore, we have the related, non-psychoactive hemp plant, which has more useful functions in textiles (clothing), fuels, rope, paper, and more, which would be a great resource for us tree-lovers. An honest reassessment of both medical marijuana and industrial hemp is long overdue so that both commodities can be used resourcefully.

Smoking marijuana can be a problematic drug habit also, and like other substances, we need to find that healthy and nondependent relationship. When it's used daily to feel high instead of dealing with emotions and life, it can be destructive. Overall, we can generally say that the least amount of drugs we use, the better.

To review, **if you have an active drug problem, stopping totally can be dangerous.** You may need a slower transition or guidance and support. Going cold turkey from sedatives, stimulants, and narcotics can have very serious consequences, including seizures. There are many doctors and facilities, such as hospital detox centers, available to help us deal with drug problems. A further discussion of and specific treatments for drug abuse are beyond the scope of this book. Many of the suggestions in this text, specifically the Detox Diet and nutritional supplement guidelines, however, can be very useful in the process of detoxifying from such destructive habits.

The nutrient program on page 208 is intended as a supplement to a medical drug detoxification program and as support during necessary drug use. The ranges given allow for varying needs. During initial withdrawal, the higher levels should be used, with mid-range levels used during the three to six weeks directly following initial withdrawal. Lower ranges may provide basic support during general drug use.

DRUG DETOX SUMMARY

1. **Drink plenty of water** and consider the alkalinizing **Detox Diet** to help you transition from your habit.

2. If you are a **heavy drug user,** use the assistance of a health-care practitioner or a clinic to support your detox. Going cold turkey from sedatives, stimulants, and narcotics can

have very serious consequences, including seizures.

3. If you are **pregnant**, use medical supervision to stop using drugs. Acupuncture has a particularly good reputation for helping moms detox and for supporting full-term, healthy babies.

4. **Reduce stress in your life.** Enhance your coping strategies and support systems.

5. **Use psychological supports** that fit your value system: counseling, biofeedback, Narcotics Anonymous (NA), or behavior modification.

6. **Use supplemental nutrients** to support your body during detox. Include regular vitamin C, B vitamins, and most minerals, particularly calcium and magnesium for their calming effects.

7. Try **herbal therapies** to ease the detox process—white willow bark for pain, valerian root and others for anxiety and insomnia. If these are not strong enough, prescription medications can be used temporarily to help ease withdrawal.

8. Consider the use of **acupuncture** and Chinese herbal therapy to ease the body through its transition.

9. Instead of reaching outwardly for a substance or other crutch, **practice breathing or a calming exercise** and then relaxation will often follow.

10. **Exercise** programs with aerobics and weights, or even yoga and qi gong, will support most detox programs.

Endnotes

1. E.J. Frech and M.F. Go, "Treatment and Chemoprevention of NSAID-Associated Gastrointestinal Complications," *Therapeutics and Clinical Risk Management* 5, no. 1 (February 2009): 65–73; R. Bystrianyk, "More Hospitalized from NSAID Bleeding Than All American War Casualties," *Health Sentinel* January 2010. www.healthsentinel.com/joomla/index .php? option=com_content&view=article&id= 266:more-hospitalized-from-nsaid-bleeding-than-all-american-war-casualties&catid=5: original&Itemid=24 (accessed November 26, 2011).

2. Brian Hoyle, "All about Aspirin," Everyday Health, www.everydayhealth.com/headache-migraine/all-about-aspirin.aspx (accessed November 26, 2011).

3. National Drug Intelligence Center, "Heroin Fast Facts," www.justice.gov/ndic/pubs3/3843/ index.htm (2003 most current found).

4. Jennifer Lloyd, "Heroin," *Almanac of Policy Issues.* www.policyalmanac.org/crime/archive/ heroin.shtml (accessed November 26, 2011).

CHAPTER FIFTEEN

Nontoxic Living

NOW THAT WE'VE TALKED ABOUT cleaning up our diet and our body, how do we decrease toxicity in our home and in the lives of all who live there? Here are some ideas for effective cleaning supplies, good health in the kitchen, and safe drinking water.

THE "NEW" OLD WAY OF CLEANING

We remember our grandmothers hanging the laundry outside to dry on the clothesline rather than using the electrical dryer. She saved money and electricity this way, had more exercise, and her sheets smelled like heavenly fresh air. Now we have a chemical spray or solution for every cleaning need to make it easier, faster, or smell good (often artificially). However, the environment and our bodies become unhealthier with every use, and we end up creating new chemical compounds when numerous chemicals are mixed. We don't know how these new chemicals will affect us in the future or how much our bodies are suffering now because of our exposure to them. In the long run, the people and the environment lose and the chemical companies win (only, however, if we consider mere money as winning).

The good news is that we are not dependent on these synthetic chemically-based products. In fact, there are many natural solutions for good cleaning. There are natural and nontoxic ways to get the same results you would achieve with standard chemical cleaning products. For example, most people think of Drano when their sinks become clogged, but it is extremely toxic to your body, the pipes, and to the environment. Instead you could use a snake (a long piece of equipment) to clean out your drain. You may be surprised at how effective it is, and you'll save money in the long run. In many cases, vinegar and baking soda poured in equal parts down the drain, followed by a plunger, will also unclog a slow-draining sink or tub. If the clog hasn't created an emergency, there are new liquids containing active enzymes that with a few days use will digest and clear the debris in the drains. I have used this in recent years with good success.

Another example of a nontoxic cleaning alternative is for your microwave when it has food odors that won't go away. Rather than use harsh cleaning sprays, squeeze half a lemon into a cup of water and just wipe the microwave with the lemon water to freshen it up. The lemon acids help cut grease if the microwave needs some cleaning as well.

Avoid antibacterial soaps and cleansers, which are harsh and add to the problem of antibiotic-resistant organisms. Some chemicals we use daily in our homes are not all that toxic on their own, but once they come into contact with other chemicals they can turn into more toxic chemical compounds. For example, when chlorine bleach combines with ammonia it forms a deadly gas. There are so many effective natural cleaning products available today that there is no reason to continue using toxic formulas. There are many books and websites that offer these natural products, as well as your local grocer or natural foods store.

A HEALTHIER KITCHEN

With a few simple changes in kitchen equipment and how you care for them, you will be able to reduce contact with synthetic materials and considerably reduce your chemical exposure overall. Here are some specific ideas:

- In the **microwave**, avoid plasticware and use glass bowls or any safe, microwavable containers. When food is heated in plastics, some of the plastic material ends up in the food, especially if the food contains acids (such as tomatoes or lemons). Glass does not leach anything into the food and is a much safer choice. Also, make sure that any ceramic you use for preparing or serving food is nontoxic and does not contain lead. Some heirloom and imported ceramics and dishes may not be food-safe because they may contain lead, arsenic, or other toxic metals.

- **Kitchen tools**, such as pots and pans that we use daily, can make a big difference in our toxic load. Avoid non-clad aluminum and use only aluminum coated with stainless steel, such as All-Clad, Calphalon, and Cuisinart cookware, stainless steel pans such as Revere Ware, or cast-iron skillets.

- **Use a preseasoned iron skillet** and it is ready to cook with, or buy an unseasoned skillet and season it yourself. This involves coating the skillet with oil that has a high smoke point, such as extra virgin olive oil, then heating the skillet at 350°F for an hour to create a nonstick coating that is left on the skillet. To maintain the coating, which creates a barrier between the cookware and your food, simply wash with hot water but without soap. Cast-iron skillets are now available in various sizes online and in many grocery stores. A small 8-inch skillet is a perfect size for single servings.

- **Pots and pans** made from stainless steel are nontoxic because they do not leach metals into food. But stainless steel alone doesn't conduct heat evenly; therefore, aluminum and copper cores ensure that foods cook evenly, without hot spots and with quick response when you turn up the heat. Some brands, such as All-Clad and Cuisinart, have a copper core to help conduct the heat evenly, and aluminum interior layers make them lighter and easier to handle. By using aluminum on the interior rather than exposed surfaces, we can have the benefits of aluminum without the exposure to the toxic metal.

- If you have **nonstick pots or pans**, be sure to use high-temperature-rated plastic or wood utensils so you don't scrape the nonstick coating (such as Teflon) into your food. Once the cookware has been scratched, it will begin to peel and bits of it end up in the food cooked on that surface. The Teflon, when heated at medium to high temperatures, releases toxic chemicals implicated in female infertility, low sperm count, and thyroid disease. Avoiding Teflon pans is the best choice. If you do have unscratched pans, only use them over low heat.[1] The greatest exposure to these dangerous chemicals come from the fast-food wrappings and the inside of microwave popcorn bags.[2]

- **Pressure cookers** allow you to cook nutritious whole foods (such as cooking beans) quickly and efficiently. The Kuhn Rikon pressure cooker is my favorite. For low-fat cooking, the bamboo steamer is the ultimate tool. Also having a blender for smoothies, a small food processor for grinding flaxseed, nuts, and herbs, and a mortar and pestle to grind spices, which releases their natural oils, gives you more freedom in preparing healthy foods.

- A **garlic press** is a must if you love fresh garlic. The Zyliss Susi garlic press works exceptionally well. Also the rubber garlic tubes sold in kitchen stores work well to remove the garlic skin. A high-quality **rubber spatula** will help you get that last drop out of jars. OXO makes high-temperature-resistance spatulas.

- A **tea ball** allows you to sample a wider variety of teas because so many come in loose form rather than in bags.

- Having a few different **cutting boards** is a good idea, one for meats and one for produce. Wood is best, and I also like my bamboo cutting boards. Rinse the produce board regularly and pour boiling water over the meat board or run it through the dishwasher frequently. And never cut other food on the same board you've cut raw chicken on without washing it first.

- **Reducing our toxin exposure** from our daily routine can make a big difference in our total body load over time. Because many of us use teapots daily to heat water for coffee or tea, they are also an important consideration. Stainless steel is fine, aluminum should be avoided, and glass (in the microwave) is an excellent option because it does not leach any chemical or metal compounds into the water.

NOISE POLLUTION AND ELECTROMAGNETIC TOXICITY

What we receive in our body comes from many things and areas of life. We have chemicals and junk food, relationship hassles, fragrances and smells, and many other forms of pollution around us all the time. We have many mouths through which we receive energy—the main mouth for food and drink; the eyes for what we see; the heart for what we feel; and the ears for what we hear. We can be polluted and affected by all of these areas of intake.

When we talk about detoxification, this covers all areas of life. Do we need to give our eyes and minds a break from all the bad news on TV every day? Do we also need breaks from the computer and other devices? And what about all the noises in our lives? We need mini-vacations and breaks from everything on occasion.

WATER PURIFICATION

Clean water is our most basic need. You can filter water at your kitchen tap with either a reverse osmosis or a solid-carbon activated charcoal filter and use it for all of your drinking water, cooking, and pets as well. You can also purchase a "solid" carbon filter system to remove metals and microbes from your home tap water.

The international bottled waters such as Perrier (France) and Evian (New Zealand) are high-quality clean waters. The regulations for bottling water in Europe are very strict, and the water is tested for contamination at the source as it is being bottled each hour. In the States, opt for local spring waters bottled in glass—try a variety to see what you like best. Also, I choose the sparkling waters bottled in glass rather than plastic. These carbonated waters are generally bubbly because of the addition of CO_2, which is safe and easy for our bodies to handle. However, sugared sodas, such as colas, are carbonated along with the addition of phosphoric acid, and excess phosphorous can have negative health effects. Phosphorous reduces calcium absorption into the bone and contributes to bone loss, which can lead to osteoporosis.

The bottled waters mentioned do not contain anything but pure water, minerals, and possibly CO_2 or natural fruit flavors. They contain no calories and are tasty soda alternatives. See *Staying Healthy with Nutrition* for more detailed health information on water. *Note:* Please realize that water stored in plastic bottles that may contain BPA should not be your main source of drinking water.

Keep bubbly water on hand and add pomegranate or orange juice to make a festive drink, or use the sparkling water in place of tonic water, which has a surprising amount of sugar in it.

CHEMICAL-FREE CLOTHING

There are many companies nowadays that promote natural fibers and organic materials. One popular one is Patagonia (www.patagonia.com), which converted their sportswear line to 100 percent organically grown cotton in 1996.[3] Cotton is one of the most heavily treated (with insecticides) crops in the United States. Ten percent of all agricultural chemicals in the United States are used to produce cotton.

Conventionally grown cotton fields in California alone are dusted every year with 6.9 million pounds of chemicals. Organic cotton is especially important for those with sensitive skin, babies, and the elderly. Even Walmart has some clothing made from organic cotton.

Some interesting facts to consider:

- Conventional cotton farming accounts for 25 percent of the world's insecticide use and more than 10 percent of the pesticides used globally, and the pesticides used on cotton are some of the most toxic. To grow enough cotton for a single T-shirt, $\frac{1}{3}$ pound of pesticides and fertilizers are used. Seventy percent of the cotton grown in the United States comes from GMO seeds.[4]

- Children and pregnant women are at greater risk for pesticide-related health problems and millions of American children already receive their lifetime dose of some carcinogenic pesticides by age five.

In addition to organic cotton, natural fibers such as hemp and linen are generally made from plants that are organically grown and untreated with chemicals. They are made into fabrics and clothing and are available on the Internet and in stores.

NATURAL CLEANING PRODUCTS

As mentioned, this is an important area for all of us who live on planet Earth to consider, because we all contribute to pollution by the cleaning and laundering choices we make in our homes. There are many companies, and more entering this area of commerce, that are conscientious and caring about the quality of products they sell. The argument for switching to more natural cleaning supplies is not just helpful to the environment; it's also important to individual health. People with respiratory problems or allergies may be particularly sensitive to fumes and fragrances in cleaning products. Many good "green" cleaning solutions use baking soda, lemon, vinegar, borax, and other common kitchen items.[5]

Learn how to create a healthy kitchen, use safe drinking water, read food labels, and find out how to avoid the chemicals that get into our food supply. Some useful online resources are the 2008 archive Fox News story "How Green Are Eco-Friendly Cleaning Products?," the World Watch Institute's article on the decline of bottled water, the Organic Consumers Association (www.organicconsumers.org) for current updates on organic agriculture, and the wonderful website EcoMom.com, which offers a variety of eco-friendly and organic food and products for the home and kids.[6]

Endnotes

1. Leah Zerbe, "Thyroid Disease Linked to Chemical in Your Kitchen," www.rodale.com/nonstick-cookware-and-teflon-dangers (accessed November 26, 2011).

2. Ibid.

3. www.patagonia.com/us/patagonia.go?assetid=2077 (accessed November 26, 2011).

4. About Organic Cotton.org, "Organic Cotton Is Different," www.aboutorganiccotton.org/OCdiff.html (accessed November 26, 2011).

5. Lisa Farino, "The Dangers Under Your Sink," MSN Health & Fitness, February 23, 2011. http://health.msn.com/health-topics/the-dangers-under-your-sink (accessed November 26, 2011).

6. Steven Kotler, "How Green Are Eco-Friendly Cleaning Products?" Fox News, January 3, 2008. www.foxnews.com/story/0,2933,318832,00.html (accessed November 26, 2011); Ben Block, "Bottled Water Demand May Be Declining," World Watch Institute. www.worldwatch.org/node/5878 (accessed November 26, 2011).

Part Three

THE
RECIPES

We have expanded the recipe options from the original version of *The Detox Diet* because we want to give you more tasty choices for foods you can consume during and after detox. The following recipes are examples of foods you can eat coming off your detox program as well as some you can even consume while on your detox. We have organized them into breakfast; lunch and dinner; soups, salads, and side dishes; sauces, dips and dressings; snacks and treats; hot and cold drinks; smoothies; and fresh vegetable and fruit juices for easier access and application to your diet.

Part of the detoxification process is following an alkaline diet to help balance the acidic body state, which we believe leads to the toxicity and inflammation that results in the chronic, degenerative problems many Westerners experience. (See the earlier discussion on the acid-alkaline balance in chapter 2.) Therefore, our program focuses on the alkaline-generating fruits and vegetables and the most alkaline grains, which include millet, quinoa, and buckwheat. We have avoided the use of commonly reactive foods, such as wheat and dairy products other than an occasional optional ingredient, as with the cheese in the Stuffed Bell Peppers (page 228).

We also suggest minimizing all chemical exposure, both from your environment and from your foods. Therefore, we support your inclusion of organic food choices whenever these are available, as well as avoiding packaged and processed foods as much as possible and minimizing chemical use at home. A review of chemical concerns and the most important foods to buy organically grown can be found in *Staying Healthy with Nutrition*.

Good appetite. Good food. Good health.

COOKING VEGETABLES

Before you go into the specific recipes, here are some general guidelines for cooking vegetables because they are so important to the whole process of detoxification. Focusing our diet around vegetables is a long-range health activity. (In fact, I have an entire cookbook devoted to this, called *More Vegetables, Please!*) The fresher the vegetables, the better, with organic the best choice to avoid toxic chemical sprays. Cooking vegetables can make these nutritious foods easier to digest for many, but cooking can also destroy many of the health-generating vitamins and minerals. It's important not to overcook vegetables. When steaming, allow the veggies to still have a little crunch. Furthermore, the liquid under the steamed veggies may be quite nutritious and helps alkalinize and rebalance the body and help fight many chronic problems.

Next, you will find healthy ways to prepare vegetables besides eating them raw and fresh. The methods described here are steaming, roasting, and water sauté. Eat a variety of four to six veggies per dish, using one or two root vegetables only, a few less-starchy vegetables like zucchini and green beans, and some leafy greens.

Steaming

For detoxifying purposes, this is the best way to prepare vegetables. After steaming, vegetables are easy to digest and still nutritious. Simply chop your veggies into appropriate sizes for eating. Use a vegetable steamer in a large pot with a few inches of water below, or invest in a double pot with the water below and the veggies above, or use an electric steamer. Start the steaming with the vegetables that take the longest time to cook; these are the hard squashes, potatoes, and roots such as carrots and beets. After 5 to 10 minutes, add the next set of veggies, such as green beans, broccoli, onions, zucchini, and the stems of chard. Finally, just before you turn off the heat, add any leafy greens to the top. Serve with Better Butter (page 235), a splash of olive oil, and the seasonings of your choice, such as sea salt, garlic salt, cayenne pepper, or other herbs. Also, save the steam water to use in drinks and soups.

Roasting

To roast vegetables, preheat the oven to 325° to 350°F (even lower will work, it just takes longer). Cut up the vegetables into edible strips or bite-size pieces. Slice zucchini and carrots lengthwise into quarters, cut potatoes into bite-size pieces, and cut mushrooms or onions into quarters. Place all in a large bowl and pour in 1 to 2 tablespoons of olive oil and mix with your hands. Sprinkle on a little vegetable salt, or Bragg's Liquid Aminos and a splash of balsamic vinegar. Place in a baking pan or dish and put in the oven. After 20 minutes or so when they are browning, take out and flip the vegetables over, and cook another 10 minutes, until they are golden brown. You can also broil for a couple of minutes at the end to add to the browning; just watch that they don't burn. Add other seasonings, if desired, before serving.

Water Sauté

Begin with a hot skillet or wok and then add a splash of olive oil to the pan along with the first layer of vegetables. (As with steaming, start with the ones needing the most cooking time and add as you go.) As the veggies cook, add small amounts of water to keep them moist. Some vegetable stock/broth or a touch of wine can also be used for more flavoring. At the end, add the leafy greens, turn off the heat, and cover for a few minutes.

Note: As with all the vegetable combinations, use the best of the seasonally available choices. These usually have the best prices and because they are local,

---

SEASONALLY AVAILABLE VEGETABLES

Spring
Artichokes, asparagus, beets and beet greens, Brussels sprouts, chard, garlic, green onions, leeks, spinach, and wild greens.

Summer
Beets and beet greens, corn, eggplant, new potatoes, peppers, soft squashes like yellow and zucchini, and sugar snap peas.

Autumn
Bell peppers, broccoli, cauliflower, celery, corn, hard squashes (acorn, butternut, spaghetti, and so on), Jerusalem artichokes, okra, potatoes, spinach, and zucchini.

Winter
Bok choy, broccoli, cabbage, cauliflower, chard, Jerusalem artichokes, kale, hard squashes, onions, potatoes, and sweet potatoes or yams.

often have less treatment with chemicals. If you buy organic, there is less concern here. Shopping at local farmers' markets when available is a great option.

ADDING PROTEIN TO VEGETABLES

When you get down to a healthier long-term diet, adding some protein, such as fish or poultry, to vegetable dishes is a healthy way to eat for energy, weight, and good health. For vegetarians, this can be beans/legumes and some nuts or seeds eaten along with the vegetables.

Begin with the appropriate amount of food you need for the number of people you wish to serve. Following a good diet means having foods available for you on a consistent basis. Therefore, even if you primarily eat alone, when you prepare nice dishes like these, make enough for two, three, or even four meals. You could use salmon, snapper, sea bass, or halibut, or buy a few turkey or chicken breasts. Also choose your favorite vegetables (hopefully you have many), primarily seasonally available ones as well as a mixture of low-starch ones as described previously. Some good ones to prepare with your proteins are onions, potatoes, carrots, zucchini, and mushrooms. A little white wine can be used as well as seasonings like olive oil, sea salt, soy sauce, garlic, and lemon.

Sauté or Pan Cooking

You can pre-marinate the strips of poultry or fish in some olive oil, tamari or sea salt, lemon, and choice of other seasonings. To a large iron skillet or wok over medium to high heat, sauté the fish or poultry on both sides for a few minutes, and then add the vegetables as you go, the firmer ones to start. (Sometimes, I put firmer veggies in first or with the protein. These are usually the garlic, onions, or mushrooms.) Cover the skillet for 5 to 10 minutes to allow the dish to cook throughout and merge its flavors. You may need to add a bit of water as you go to keep it moist.

There are many flavoring options for these dishes. Here are some general guidelines for flavoring:

- For Asian tastes, try soy sauce, ginger, and cayenne or chile.

- For Mexican flavors, use tomato, onion, cilantro, and of course, chile or cayenne peppers.

- For Mediterranean tastes, add olive oil, garlic, marjoram, rosemary, and thyme.

Baking Dish Method

Preheat the oven to 350°F. Place the fish or poultry in the baking dish, adding the appropriate seasonings, such as lemon, sea salt, garlic, and olive oil for the fish, or salt and herbs for the poultry. Cover and surround with the vegetables. You can use potatoes, carrots, onion, mushrooms, or

RECIPES FOR MENU PLANNING

Breakfast
Basic Steel-Cut Oatmeal
Gluten-Free Oatmeal with
    Blueberries
Hot Breakfast Quinoa
Breakfast Millet
Baked Apples
Dani's Muesli
Dr. Elson's Breakfast Rice

Lunch and Dinner
Cherry Tomato Salad and
    Ginger Dressing
Caesarless Salad
Millet Pilaf
Quick Southwest Quinoa
Herbed Millet with Steamed
    Vegetables
Quinoa Tabbouleh Salad
Stuffed Bell Peppers
Green Pea Hummus
Salmon with Roasted Garlic
    and Rosemary
Vegetable Curry
Lentil Stew

**Soups, Salads,
and Side Dishes**
Herbed Soup
Gazpacho
Kombu-Squash Soup
Broccoli Soup
Caraway Cabbage Borscht
Jicama Salad
White Bean Salad
Glazed Broccoli
Smoked Wild Salmon Salad
Asian Cucumber Salad
Basic Millet

Toasted Millet
Basic Quinoa
Caramelized Onion Quinoa

**Sauces, Dips,
and Dressings**
Better Butter
Tomato Vinaigrette
Rosemary-Citrus Dressing
Creamy Garlic Sauce
Date and Orange Chutney
Lemon and Olive Oil
    Dressing
Ginger Garlic Dressing
Avocado Dressing
Quick Spicy Tomato Sauce
Cilantro Pesto
Parsley Pesto
Mango Salsa
Dr. Elson's Savory Sauce

Snacks and Treats
Cold Almonds
Frozen Grapes
Mochi with Sauce
Fruit Salad with Dani's
    Muesli
Juice Jells
Guacamole and Vegetables
Kombu Knots
Pears in Black Cherry
    Sauce

Hot and Cold Drinks
Coffee substitutes, like Pos-
    tum, Cafix, or Teechino
Herbal teas, like pepper-
    mint, chamomile, or
    lemongrass

Rosemary Lemon Water
Apple Ginger Tea
Pellegrino and Bitters
    Cocktail
Gingered Green Tea
Cinnamon Cider
Citrus Sparkle
Cucumber and Lemon
    Water (Indian Springs
    Health Elixir)
Hibiscus Tea Cooler
Apple Lemon Spritzer

Smoothies
Ginger Cooler
Peachy Orange
Strawberry-Orange Shake
Purple Papaya
Banana Soother
Avocado Freeze
Tahini Shake
Cinnamon Pears
Tobin's Strawberry Almond
    Shake

**Fresh Vegetable
and Fruit Juices**
Carrot Cocktail
After Workout Refresher
Energizing Elixir
Cucumber Cooler
Immune Supporter
Apple Lemonade
Tropical Twist
Fresh Harvest
Sunset Soother

brussels sprouts cut in half. If I add zucchini or bell peppers or greens, I put them in about halfway through cooking. Add a splash of water if needed to keep the food moist. Cover and bake for 30 to 45 minutes. This is a full meal, yet for a more typically complete one, you can also serve with a fresh salad or some rice.

BREAKFAST

Basic Steel-Cut Oatmeal

Steel-cut oats are less processed than rolled or instant oats, so they metabolize more slowly, providing longer-lasting fuel for your body. You can add fruit to this oatmeal if you would like. SERVES 3

    3 cups water, juice, or rice or oat milk
    1/4 teaspoon salt
    1 cup steel-cut oats
    1 tablespoon maple syrup

In a saucepan, bring the water and salt to a boil over high heat. Add the steel-cut oats and return to a boil. Reduce the heat to low, cover, and cook for 10 to 20 minutes, depending on how chewy or soft you like your cereal. Remove from the heat and let stand, covered, for a couple of minutes until slightly thickened. Serve with maple syrup.

Gluten-Free* Oatmeal with Blueberries

SERVES 2

    2 cups water
    Pinch of salt
    Pinch of cardamom
    1 cup gluten-free rolled oats (such as Bob's Red Mill brand)
    1/2 cup rice milk
    1 tablespoon ground flaxseed
    2 tablespoons maple syrup
    2 tablespoons sunflower seeds
    1/2 cup blueberries

In a saucepan, bring the water, salt, and cardamom to a boil over high heat and stir in the rolled oats. Let simmer for 15 to 18 minutes, stirring occasionally. Serve with rice milk, flaxseed, a drizzle of maple syrup, sunflower seeds, and blueberries.

* Oats are typically gluten-free, but some companies are not as careful about gluten grain (wheat, rye, and barley) contamination. Other companies like Bob's Red Mill tests its oats to make sure.

Hot Breakfast Quinoa

Quinoa is delicious with toppings such as shredded coconut, raisins, and Cold Almonds (page 239). SERVES 4

1 cup quinoa

2 cups water

Salt

1/2 cup chopped apples, pears, raisins, soaked almonds, or dates (optional)

1/2 cup rice milk

1 tablespoon maple syrup

Pineapple bits, toasted shredded coconut, and/or 1/2 teaspoon cinnamon, for garnish (optional)

Rinse the quinoa under cold running water and drain. Place the quinoa in a saucepan over high heat, add the water and salt, and bring to a boil. Reduce the heat and simmer for 5 minutes. Add whatever fruit you desire, or none at all, and continue to simmer until all the water is absorbed. Serve with rice milk and a drizzle of maple syrup. Garnish with pineapple, coconut, and/or cinnamon.

Breakfast Millet

Millet will pick up the flavor of the sweetener. To add more protein and fiber to your breakfast, sprinkle the top with soaked almonds. SERVES 2

1 cup water

1/4 teaspoon salt

1/4 cup millet

1 cup rice milk

2 tablespoons maple syrup

Place the water, salt, and millet in a saucepan and cook over low heat for 25 to 30 minutes, until all of the water has been absorbed. Serve with rice milk; drizzle with maple syrup.

Baked Apples

SERVES 4

4 organic green apples

1/4 cup raisins

8 almonds

1/4 teaspoon cinnamon

2 cups water

Preheat the oven to 350°F. Wash the apples and slice 1/2 inch off the top. Set the tops aside. Core the apples with an apple corer, being careful not to puncture the bottom of the apples. Stuff each apple with 1 tablespoon raisins, 2 almonds, and a sprinkle of cinnamon. Fill each apple with water and replace the tops. Transfer the apples to a baking dish and bake for 30 to 40 minutes, or until soft.

Dani's Muesli

This fiber-rich breakfast cereal provides essential fatty acids and minerals that support detoxification. You can grind flaxseeds yourself just before preparing the recipe, or store flaxseed meal in the refrigerator until you're ready to use it. SERVES 10

2 pounds organic rolled oats

1 pound oat bran

1/2 pound lecithin granules

1/2 pound flaxseed meal

1/2 pound dried raisins or currants

4 ounces raw pumpkin seeds

4 ounces pecans

6 ounces wheat germ

1/2 cup live culture yogurt, plain unsweetened (optional)

1 piece of fruit, cut into small pieces, or 1/2 cup berries (optional)

Mix all the dry ingredients in a very large mixing bowl or a paper bag. Store in plastic bags or containers in a cool dry place. The freezer is a good place to keep a majority of the muesli. To serve, soak 1/2 to 3/4 cup of muesli for at least 30 minutes in diluted fruit juice or water. Top with the yogurt and/or fruit. If you are having digestive problems, you may want to soak the muesli in water overnight to help soften the oats further.

Tips:

- *Sweet crunchy apples are delicious with this recipe.*

- *To mix the ingredients, use the biggest mixing bowl you have or a large paper bag, or split the ingredients into two batches.*

- *Store unused muesli in your freezer in resealable plastic bags.*

Dr. Elson's Breakfast Rice

SERVES 4

1 cup raisins

1 tablespoon grated lemon zest

1 cinnamon stick or 1/2 teaspoon ground cinnamon

1 cup apple juice

4 cups cooked brown rice

1/2 cup coarsely chopped walnuts or almonds, lightly toasted

Place the raisins, lemon zest, cinnamon, and apple juice in a saucepan and simmer over low heat for 3 to 5 minutes, until the raisins are plump. Add the rice and simmer a few minutes longer, turn off the heat, add the walnuts, and let stand, covered, for 10 minutes or longer, until all the liquid is absorbed. Serve warm.

Cherry Tomato Salad and Ginger Dressing

SERVES 2

2 cups dark leafy greens, chopped

1 cup cherry tomatoes

Dressing:

2 cloves garlic

1 tablespoon fresh ginger

1 teaspoon brown mustard

1 teaspoon lemon juice

1 teaspoon balsamic vinegar

2 tablespoons walnut oil

Salt, to taste

Wash the greens and tomatoes and set aside to dry. To make the dressing, press the garlic and ginger through a garlic press into a bowl and add the rest of the ingredients. Chop the greens, then drizzle the dressing over the greens and tomatoes and toss well. Serve immediately.

Caesarless Salad

SERVES 2

2 tablespoons flaxseed oil

2 tablespoons lemon juice

2 garlic cloves, minced

1 head romaine lettuce, torn into bite-size pieces

1/4 teaspoon sea salt

1 tablespoon nutritional yeast

1/4 cup walnuts, chopped

1/4 cup sliced red bell pepper

Combine the flaxseed oil, lemon juice, and garlic in a large salad bowl. Mix well. Add the lettuce and toss until the leaves are well coated. Sprinkle salt and nutritional yeast over the lettuce and toss again. Add the walnuts and bell pepper slices and serve.

Millet Pilaf

This flavorful dish can be modified to include your favorite vegetables. For added color and flavor, try adding chopped zucchini, carrots, red peppers, or celery when you add the other fresh vegetables. SERVES 4

1 cup millet

4 cups vegetable broth or water

1 cup chopped parsley

1 tomato, chopped

1/2 cup chopped green onion

Salt and black pepper

In a saucepan over low heat, combine the millet and vegetable broth, and cook for 25 to 35 minutes, until all the broth has been absorbed. Add the parsley, tomato, and green onion. Season with salt and pepper. Serve warm or store in a covered container in the refrigerator for up to 4 days.

Quick Southwest Quinoa

Quinoa can be cooked ahead of time and kept in the refrigerator for up to 5 days. By having prepared quinoa on hand, you can whip up this dish in minutes when you don't feel like cooking. SERVES 4

2 cups cooked quinoa

1 cup fresh salsa

1/4 cup chopped cilantro

1/2 lemon or lime (optional)

Minced jalapeño or fresh chopped tomato, for garnish (optional)

In a serving bowl, combine the quinoa with the salsa and cilantro. If desired, squeeze 1/2 lemon or lime over the top for a fresh tangy addition or garnish with some jalapeño or tomato. Serve warm or cold.

Herbed Millet with Steamed Vegetables

This simple, spicy dish is versatile and a hearty accompaniment to wild salmon, a green salad, or steamed vegetables. SERVES 4

1 cup millet

2 cups vegetable broth or water

1/2 onion, finely chopped

3 small cloves garlic, minced

1 teaspoon chopped fresh sage

Combine all the ingredients in a saucepan over low heat. Cook for 30 to 40 minutes, until all the liquid has been absorbed. Serve warm.

Quinoa Tabbouleh Salad

Fresh parsley, mint, and lemon juice are the bright flavors that make this Lebanese dish so popular. The quinoa mingles beautifully with these flavors. SERVES 4

1 cup cooked quinoa

1 green onion, minced

1 1/4 cups minced parsley

1/2 cup minced fresh mint

1 tablespoon freshly squeezed lemon juice

1 tablespoon extra virgin olive oil or flaxseed oil

1 teaspoon ground cumin

Combine all the ingredients and serve immediately or chill in a covered container for up to 4 days.

Stuffed Bell Peppers

Stuffed bell peppers are a meal in themselves or serve with a green or grain salad, such as Quinoa Tabbouleh Salad (above). SERVES 4

4 green, red, or yellow bell peppers

2 teaspoons sesame oil

1 or 2 cloves garlic, minced or pressed

1 cup albacore tuna or cooked beans

2 cups cooked brown rice

2 green onions, including green parts, finely chopped

2 tablespoons chopped fresh cilantro, or 1 teaspoon ground coriander

1 to 2 tablespoons salsa

Sea salt

Freshly ground black pepper

4 tablespoons cheese (optional)

Preheat the oven to 400°F.

Cut the tops off the peppers and set the tops aside. Scoop out the seeds and ribs and discard. Combine the sesame oil, garlic, tuna, brown rice, green onion, cilantro, and salsa in a bowl. Season with salt and pepper. Stuff the peppers with the mixture. Place the peppers on a baking sheet, right side up, and replace the pepper tops. Bake for 25 minutes. Remove the tops of the bell peppers and set aside. Sprinkle each pepper with 1 tablespoon cheese and bake for 5 more minutes, until the cheese is melted. Replace the pepper tops and serve immediately.

Green Pea Hummus

This brilliant green dip is fresh, filling, and perfect for entertaining. Serve with colorful vegetable slices as an appetizer or afternoon snack. SERVES 4

2 cups fresh or frozen peas

2 cloves garlic

Juice of ½ lemon

2 tablespoons toasted tahini

Salt and freshly ground pepper

1 tablespoon ground cumin

1 tablespoon extra virgin olive oil (optional)

Baby carrots, celery sticks, and/or sweet red, orange, or yellow bell pepper slices, for serving

Mix the peas, garlic, lemon juice, tahini, salt and pepper, cumin, and oil in a blender or food processor until smooth. Serve in a bowl with baby carrots, celery sticks, and/or sliced bell pepper.

Salmon with Roasted Garlic and Rosemary

This salmon is also great cooked on the grill. SERVES 4

2 bulbs garlic, unpeeled

3 tablespoons freshly squeezed lemon juice

4 sprigs fresh rosemary, or 1 teaspoon dried

¼ cup extra virgin olive oil

2 (8- to 10-ounce) wild salmon fillets

Preheat the oven to 350°F. Wrap the garlic bulbs loosely in aluminum foil and lay directly on the oven rack. Roast the garlic for 45 minutes, or until the cloves are very tender when tested with a knife. Remove the garlic from the oven and let cool. Peel the garlic, discarding the outer skin. In a food processor, combine the garlic, lemon juice, rosemary, and oil. Puree until smooth. Spread the puree on the salmon. Lightly oil the baking dish with extra virgin olive oil. Transfer the salmon to the baking dish and bake until flaky, about 20 to 30 minutes.

Vegetable Curry

Ghee (a type of clarified butter that originated in India) and asafetida (a flavoring used in Indian dishes) can be found in Indian markets, some grocery stores, or online. SERVES 4 TO 6

1 large butternut squash

2 tablespoons ghee

1 tablespoon curry powder

$\frac{1}{2}$ teaspoon ground cardamom

$\frac{1}{2}$ teaspoon ground cumin

$\frac{1}{2}$ teaspoon ground coriander

$\frac{1}{2}$ teaspoon ground ginger

$\frac{1}{2}$ teaspoon asafetida (optional)

$\frac{1}{2}$ teaspoon anise seed

$\frac{1}{2}$ teaspoon turmeric

2 small onions, sliced

2 carrots, sliced diagonally

1 small cauliflower, cut into florets

1 cup green beans, cut into 2-inch lengths

2 cups water

Sea salt

$\frac{1}{3}$ cup tahini

4 cups cooked basmati rice

Cut the butternut squash in half, remove the seeds, and cut into pieces, leaving the skin on. Transfer the squash to a large pot with water almost to cover, and boil until the pieces can be pierced with a fork. Transfer the squash to a blender or food processor and blend until pureed. Set aside.

In a heavy-bottomed saucepan, add the ghee, spices, and onion. Sauté over medium-low heat, stirring frequently, until the onion is limp and the spices are fragrant. Add the carrots, sauté a few minutes, add the cauliflower, sauté a few minutes longer, and then add the beans. Add the water and season with salt; cover, and simmer for 15 minutes. Add the tahini and pureed squash, and cook, stirring, until heated through. Serve over the basmati rice.

Lentil Stew

SERVES 4

1 cup raw lentils

2 large carrots, thinly sliced

2 stalks celery, chopped

1 large onion, chopped

3 to 5 cloves garlic, crushed

1 tablespoon olive oil

1 (14-ounce) can Italian tomatoes

$\frac{1}{4}$ teaspoon ground cumin

1 teaspoon coriander seeds

$\frac{1}{2}$ teaspoon salt

$\frac{1}{4}$ teaspoon black pepper

3 tablespoons balsamic vinegar

In a saucepan over medium heat, combine all the ingredients and cook for 30 minutes, until soft.

Herbed Soup

SERVES 8

10 cloves garlic, minced

$1/2$ cup chopped Italian parsley or cilantro

2 bay leaves

1 teaspoon dried sage

5 whole cloves

Pinch of dried thyme

2 quarts vegetable broth

$1/4$ teaspoon freshly ground black pepper

1 (14-ounce) can stewed tomatoes

1 (16-ounce) can white beans, rinsed and
    drained

Sea salt

Pinch of saffron threads

Freshly squeezed lime or lemon juice, to taste
    (optional)

Place the garlic, parsley, bay leaves, sage, cloves, thyme, broth, pepper, tomatoes, beans, and salt in a large stockpot over high heat and bring to a boil. Stir well, cover, reduce the heat, and simmer for 30 minutes. While the soup is cooking, dry-roast the saffron: Heat a skillet over low heat. Add the saffron gently and stir constantly for 3 minutes to release the oils. Just before the soup is finished, add the saffron to the soup, stirring to combine. Remove the soup from the heat, and let stand for 5 minutes. Squeeze the lime juice over the top. Serve warm.

Gazpacho

This cold soup is not cooked and is therefore considered raw food. It is rich in antioxidants. SERVES 6 TO 8

1 cup finely chopped red onion

2 cups seeded and finely chopped cucumber

1 cup seeded and finely diced green bell
    pepper

1 cup seeded and finely chopped red bell
    pepper

1 (28-ounce) can tomato puree

3 cloves garlic, minced

$1/4$ cup rice wine vinegar

$1/4$ fresh jalapeño pepper, minced

$1/2$ teaspoon freshly ground black pepper

$1/4$ cup dry red wine or balsamic vinegar

$1/4$ cup water

1 tablespoon freshly squeezed lime juice

3 tablespoons freshly squeezed lemon juice

1 cup finely chopped fresh cilantro

Combine all the ingredients in a large container and chill for at least 20 minutes. This cold soup can be refrigerated in an airtight container for up to 5 days. Serve chilled.

Kombu-Squash Soup

This is a great autumn-winter alkalizing and warming soup. SERVES 10

6 cups water

4 cups chopped butternut squash

1 (8-inch) piece kombu

1 tablespoon extra virgin olive oil

1 large onion, chopped

4 cloves garlic, minced

2-inch-long piece ginger, chopped

1/4 cup balsamic vinegar

Sea salt

Bring the water to a boil in a large saucepan over high heat. Add the squash and the kombu, reduce the heat to medium, and cook for 20 minutes. Remove the squash from the saucepan and cut away the skin. Discard the skin and return the squash to the saucepan.

In a skillet, heat the olive oil over medium heat. Add the onion, garlic, and ginger and sauté for about 10 minutes. Add the sautéed vegetables to the squash mixture and cook for 1 hour, until the squash is tender. Stir in the balsamic vinegar, season with salt, and serve.

Broccoli Soup

SERVES 4

1 (14-ounce) can vegetable or chicken broth

2 cups water

1 pound broccoli, chopped

1 cup sliced carrots

1 onion, sliced into rings

1 teaspoon salt

1/2 to 1 teaspoon coarsely ground black pepper (optional)

Combine the broth and water in a saucepan over high heat. Bring to a boil and add the broccoli, carrots, and onion. Season with salt and pepper. Simmer for about 30 minutes, or until the vegetables are tender. For a creamier soup, blend briefly in a blender or food processor.

Caraway Cabbage Borscht

SERVES 4 TO 6

2 tablespoons extra virgin olive oil

2 large yellow onions, chopped

1 carrot, sliced

1 stalk celery, chopped

4 cups shredded cabbage

4 beets, cut into matchsticks

2 tablespoons caraway seeds

2 teaspoons salt

Freshly ground black pepper (optional)

4 cups water

1 (6-ounce) can tomato paste

2 tablespoons apple cider vinegar

1 tablespoon maple syrup

1 teaspoon dill (optional)

In a large soup pot, heat the olive oil over medium heat. Add the onions and stir over medium-high heat until caramelized. Add the carrot, celery, cabbage, beets, caraway seeds, salt, and pepper and stir well. Add the water and tomato paste and continue to cook over medium heat for 20 minutes longer. Add the vinegar, maple syrup, and dill. Serve warm or cold, or store in a glass container in the refrigerator for up to 4 days.

Jicama Salad

SERVES 4

1 jicama, grated

1 carrot, grated

1/2 cup fresh basil leaves

1/8 to 1/4 jalapeño pepper, grated

1/4 cup chopped mint leaves

1 tablespoon freshly squeezed lime juice

Toss all the ingredients together in a large bowl. Serve immediately.

White Bean Salad

SERVES 4

1 (12-ounce) can white beans, rinsed and drained

1 cup chopped fresh Italian parsley

2 tomatoes, chopped

1/2 red onion, minced

1/2 lemon

2 tablespoons balsamic vinegar

1/4 teaspoon sea salt

In a large bowl, mix all the ingredients and serve, or store, covered, in the refrigerator for up to 4 days.

Glazed Broccoli

SERVES 4

2 cups chopped broccoli

1 medium red onion, thinly sliced

1 tablespoon rice vinegar or balsamic vinegar

1 tablespoon brown mustard

1 tablespoon maple syrup

In a large skillet over medium heat, steam the broccoli and onion in about 1 inch of water for 10 minutes, until tender. In a small bowl, combine the vinegar, mustard, and maple syrup. Pour the maple glaze over the vegetables, and stir until evenly coated. Serve as a side dish or over cooked quinoa or rice and/or with fish.

Smoked Wild Salmon Salad

Wild salmon is a rich source of healthy oils such as omega-3 fatty acids. Crumble over salads or cooked grains. Eat alone or drizzle with one of the dressings. SERVES 2

4 cups salad greens

2 cups cooked quinoa, rice, or millet

1/2 pound wild smoked salmon

2 to 3 tablespoons Ginger Garlic Dressing (page 237) or Creamy Garlic Sauce (page 236)

Place the greens in a bowl, add the cooked grains, crumble the salmon over, and top with a few tablespoons of dressing.

Asian Cucumber Salad

Tobin Jutte developed this recipe while participating in one of Daniella's detox workshops. After drinking his Indian Springs Cucumber Lemon Water, he found that the crisp cucumber slices could be made into a salad. SERVES 1

  1 cucumber, peeled and sliced
  1 tablespoon chopped red bell pepper
  ¼ cup rice wine vinegar
  ¼ cup water
  1 tablespoon maple syrup
  Pinch of five-spice powder and cayenne
    pepper (optional)

Combine all the ingredients in a bowl, let stand for 15 minutes, and serve.

Basic Millet

This grain has a light delicate flavor that takes on the character of whatever it is cooked with. SERVES 2

  1 cup millet, toasted or plain
  2 cups water, juice, or vegetable broth
  Salt

In a saucepan over low heat, add the water and millet and cook for 25 to 35 minutes, until the liquid has been absorbed. Season with salt.

Toasted Millet

SERVES 2

  1 cup millet

In a dry skillet over medium heat, add the millet and cook, stirring, for 6 minutes, until the grains turn a light golden brown. Be careful not to over-cook. Toasted millet can be stored for up to 2 days in the refrigerator before cooking, but it is better if used immediately.

Basic Quinoa

Quinoa is a versatile grain that can be used in place of rice with a stir-fry. Many people choose quinoa because it is higher in protein and provides longer-lasting energy than higher-carbohydrate grains. SERVES 2

  2 cups water, juice, or vegetable broth
  1 cup quinoa
  Salt

Place the water and quinoa in a 2-quart saucepan and bring to a boil. Reduce to a simmer, cover, and cook until all the water is absorbed, 15 to 20 minutes. The grain should appear translucent and the germ ring will be visible. Quinoa can be toasted before cooking to give it a nutty flavor (you can toast almost any grain before cooking). To toast, place the grain in a hot, dry skillet over medium-high heat, stirring until it is golden brown. Be careful not to over-toast the grain. Some of the grains will "pop" during toasting, so be prepared for these hot flying missiles.

Caramelized Onion Quinoa

SERVES 2

1 tablespoon extra virgin olive oil
½ cup chopped onion
⅓ cup quinoa
⅔ cup water

Add the oil and onion to a hot skillet and sauté for 5 minutes. Rinse the quinoa and add to the skillet. Add the water and bring to a boil. Reduce to a simmer and continue to cook for 10 to 15 minutes, or until all the water is absorbed. Serve warm as a side dish or with vegetables.

Better Butter

Better Butter is healthier than butter alone because it is made with half olive or flaxseed oil, so the combination has more monosaturated fats and half the saturated fat and half the cholesterol of butter. YIELDS 2 CUPS

1 cup organic extra virgin olive oil or flaxseed oil
1 cup (2 sticks) organic butter, at room temperature

Combine the olive oil and butter in a glass bowl, whip together by hand, and store, covered, in the refrigerator for up to 2 weeks.

Lemon and Olive Oil Dressing

This light dressing is the perfect finish for summer salads. SERVES 4

Juice of 1 lemon
¼ cup extra-virgin olive oil
Sea salt to taste

Whisk together the lemon juice, olive oil, and salt. Use to dress a salad. Or you can simplify the process and sprinkle each ingredient onto your salad separately, then toss the salad well.

Ginger Garlic Dressing

SERVES 8

½ orange

2-inch-long piece fresh ginger

5 cloves garlic

2 tablespoons balsamic vinegar

2 tablespoons extra virgin olive oil

Juice of ¼ lemon

1 tablespoon tamari soy sauce,
    or ½ teaspoon sea salt (optional)

Peel the orange by cutting off just the outside bright orange part of the peel, leaving the inner white pithy part, which contains all of its beneficial bioflavonoids. Combine all the ingredients in a blender and blend for 30 to 60 seconds. If you prefer a creamier dressing, blend longer. To thin the dressing, add a tablespoon of water and blend again until smooth. Serve over leafy greens, steamed vegetables, grains, or fish.

Avocado Dressing

SERVES 4

2 medium avocados, peeled and pitted

Juice of 1 lemon

1 teaspoon salt or tamari

½ cup water

⅛ teaspoon cayenne pepper

1 clove garlic (more, if desired)

Puree all the ingredients in a blender and toss with leafy greens.

Note: The following four sauces are fat free (made without oils). This is helpful for those looking for lower-calorie or low-fat diets. Even though good vegetable oils, especially monounsaturated fats, are healthy for us, we may wish to keep our calories and fats lower during detox.

Tomato Vinaigrette

YIELDS 1 CUP

Juice of ½ lemon

1 tablespoon balsamic vinegar

1 small clove garlic, minced

½ teaspoon Dijon mustard

¼ teaspoon dried thyme

¼ teaspoon dried marjoram

1 large tomato, peeled and seeded

Sea salt

In a food processor or blender, combine all the ingredients. Serve over seasonal mixed greens.

Rosemary-Citrus Dressing

SERVES 4

3 tablespoons freshly squeezed lemon juice

3 tablespoons tamari

2 tablespoons flaxseed oil

2 tablespoons fresh rosemary, chopped

Place all the ingredients in a covered jar and shake well. Use immediately or store in the refrigerator for up to one week.

Creamy Garlic Sauce

This is excellent over steamed vegetables, baked potatoes, or grains. YIELDS ABOUT 2 CUPS

15 cloves garlic, peeled and left whole
1/8 teaspoon dried sage
1/8 teaspoon dried thyme
1 1/2 cups water
2 tablespoons dry white wine (optional)
Juice of 1/2 lemon
Sea salt, to taste
2 tablespoons minced parsley
Cayenne pepper, to taste

In a saucepan, combine the garlic, sage, thyme, water, and wine. Simmer over low heat for 20 to 30 minutes, until the garlic is soft. Remove from the heat, transfer the mixture to a blender, and puree. Add the lemon juice and salt. Stir in the parsley and season with the cayenne. Reheat over low heat before serving.

Note: Cayenne pepper often comes in various heat levels. It is a great warming and energizing spice that is not usually irritating. People vary in their ability to enjoy it, so add to taste.

Date and Orange Chutney

SERVES 4 TO 6

1 whole orange, peeled and chopped
1 cup chopped pitted dates
1 teaspoon grated fresh ginger

1/3 cup water
1/3 cup rice vinegar
1 tablespoon brown rice syrup
1/4 cup raisins
Crushed red pepper flakes, to taste
Sea salt, to taste

Combine all the ingredients in a saucepan. Partially cover and cook over medium-low heat for 20 to 30 minutes, until soft. This chutney keeps well in the refrigerator for several weeks.

Quick Spicy Tomato Sauce

This rich sauce makes a meal hearty when served over fish, lentils, or cooked whole grains such as quinoa. YIELDS ABOUT 4 CUPS

1 tablespoon extra virgin olive oil
1 to 2 shallots or 1/2 red onion, chopped
2 cloves garlic, minced
1 tablespoon ground coriander
1 teaspoon ground cumin
1/4 teaspoon turmeric
1/2 teaspoon sea salt
3 cups chopped tomatoes

Heat the oil in a saucepan over medium heat. Add the shallot and garlic and sauté for 5 minutes, until soft. Add the coriander, cumin, turmeric, and salt and continue cooking, stirring, for a minute or longer, until the spices are fragrant and the shallot begins to brown. Stir in the tomatoes, cover, and cook gently over low heat for 15 minutes, until the tomatoes have turned to liquid.

Cilantro Pesto

This recipe is rich in phytonutrients. The cilantro contains volatile oils, which promote the elimination of mercury and other heavy metals. SERVES 2 TO 4

- 2 cups packed fresh cilantro, rinsed
- 2 cloves garlic
- 1/3 cups nuts (pumpkin seeds, walnuts, pine nuts, pecans, or toasted almonds)
- 1/2 cup extra virgin olive oil
- 2 tablespoons lemon juice
- Salt and pepper, to taste
- 1/2 teaspoon cayenne pepper (optional)

In a food processor, combine all the ingredients and blend to the desired consistency. Serve with rice crackers, over rice pasta or steamed vegetables, or as a dip with sliced raw vegetables.

Parsley Pesto

Parsley pesto is another recipe full of phytonutrients. Parsley contains detoxifying glutathione, which helps remove toxins and heavy metals from the body, as well as volatile oils that neutralize particular types of carcinogens (such as the benzopyrenes that are part of cigarette smoke and charcoal grill smoke). SERVES 2 TO 4

- 2 cups packed fresh parsley, rinsed
- 2 cloves garlic
- 1/3 cup nuts (pumpkin seeds, walnuts, pine nuts, pecans, or toasted almonds)
- 1/2 cup extra virgin olive oil

- 2 tablespoons lemon juice
- Salt and pepper, to taste
- 1/2 teaspoon cayenne pepper (optional)

In a food processor, combine all the ingredients and blend to the desired consistency. Serve with rice crackers, over rice pasta or steamed vegetables, or as a dip with sliced raw vegetables.

Mango Salsa

Jalapeño peppers can vary in strength. Some are very hot and overpower the recipe. Touch the pepper with a fork and touch your tongue to the fork. This will you give you an idea of how hot your pepper is. Adjust the amount of pepper accordingly. It is also a good idea to taste the onion before adding it. The age and type of onion will alter the intensity. If you have a particularly strong onion, just reduce the quantity. SERVES 6

- 1 mango, peeled, pitted, and minced
- 1/2 cup chopped red bell pepper
- 1/2 cup minced red onion
- 1 tablespoon minced jalapeño pepper
- 1 tablespoon minced fresh mint leaves
- 1 tablespoon balsamic vinegar
- 2 tablespoons freshly squeezed lime juice
- 1 tomato, minced (optional)

Combine all the ingredients in a medium bowl and mix thoroughly. Serve immediately or store in a covered container in the refrigerator for up to 1 week.

Dr. Elson's Savory Sauce

This can be used as a mochi dip or a sauce for grilled vegetables with rice or quinoa.

SERVES 2 TO 4

2 tablespoons almond butter or tahini

1 tablespoon organic miso paste

1 tablespoon honey

Pinch of cayenne pepper, or to taste

1 tablespoon water (or to preferred consistency)

Combine all the ingredients in a bowl and stir with a fork, adding water until you have your desired texture.

SNACKS AND TREATS

Cold Almonds

Soaking nuts helps soften their fiber, making them easier to digest. They taste fresh and cool and make an easy-to-grab snack for those on the run. This process works with all nuts, such as cashews, hazelnuts, and walnuts. SERVES 6

1 pound organic raw almonds

Filtered water

Pour the almonds into a large bowl and cover with filtered water. Soak for at least 4 hours. Keep the nuts in the water until they are eaten. Use as a snack or to top oatmeal and other cooked grains.

Frozen Grapes

SERVES 3

2 cups organic grapes

Wash the grapes and remove from the stem. (If there are seeds, eating some is healthful.) Pat the grapes dry and place them in a ziptop bag in the freezer. Frozen grapes make the perfect snack on hot days and are a nice addition to fruit or green salads, or as ice cubes in drinks.

Mochi with Sauce

SERVES 4

1 (17-ounce) package mochi

Honey, Better Butter (page 235), nut butter, or maple syrup (optional)

Mochi is essentially compressed, cooked, brown rice. It is sold in a variety of sweet and savory flavors. Follow the directions for baking listed on the package. As the mochi bakes it rises, forming a pastry that is chewy on the inside and crunchy on the outside—simple and yet so decadent. The cinnamon mochi begs for a dab of Better Butter and a drizzle of honey or maple syrup to serve as a dessert or with tea. The savory flavors can be served as part of a meal or as a snack and can be filled with garlic sautéed in Better Butter, or with a bit of Dr. Elson's Savory Sauce (see above).

Fruit Salad with Dani's Muesli

SERVES 1

½ cup dark berries (blueberries or blackberries)

½ cup apple, banana, or other favorite fruit

¼ to ½ cup Dani's Muesli (page 226)

¼ cup organic yogurt (optional)

Wash the berries and place them in a bowl. Add the chopped apple and top with the muesli and yogurt. This high-fiber, antioxidant-rich treat makes a hearty snack or a refreshing breakfast alternative.

Juice Jells

SERVES 4

2 cups fresh fruit juice (apple, berry, cranberry, grape, and so on)

1 to 2 teaspoons agar

Combine the juice and agar flakes in a saucepan and let stand for 2 to 3 minutes. Bring the juice to a simmer over low heat and cook, stirring, for about 10 minutes, until the agar is dissolved. Continue stirring the mixture over low heat for 5 minutes longer. Transfer to serving dishes and chill in the refrigerator for at least 2 hours, until thickened. Serve cold or frozen as ice pops.

Guacamole and Vegetables

SERVES 4

2 ripe medium to large avocados, peeled, pitted, and minced

2 ripe small to medium tomatoes, minced

3 cloves garlic, minced or 1 teaspoon garlic powder

3 tablespoons freshly squeezed lemon or lime juice

1 teaspoon balsamic vinegar

¼ red onion, minced

4 cups sliced raw vegetables, such as baby carrots, zucchini slices, and orange, red, and yellow bell peppers

In a serving bowl, mash the avocados, tomatoes, garlic, lemon juice, vinegar, and onion together using a fork. Serve with the crunchy vegetables.

Kombu Knots

Kombu is naturally salty and lends just the right flavor to this potato chip–like snack. Seaweeds help alkalinize the body. SERVES 4 TO 8

1 (2-ounce) package kombu

Extra virgin olive oil, for cooking

Soak the kombu in water to soften. Using scissors, cut the kombu into strips about ⅛ inch wide and 3 inches long. Tie the strips into simple knots. Pour the oil into a small saucepan to a depth of up to 1 inch. Set over medium-high heat until the oil is hot, but not smoking. Drop the kombu knots into the oil, making sure they are submerged, and cook for about 1 minute each. Transfer to a paper towel to drain.

Pears in Black Cherry Sauce

SERVES 4

- 4 firm pears
- 2-inch-long piece fresh ginger, cut into matchsticks, or 1 tablespoon grated fresh ginger
- 4 cups black cherry juice
- 3 tablespoons kudzu dissolved in ¼ cup cold water
- 4 sprigs mint, for garnish

Place the pears and ginger in a large, heavy-bottomed pot and add the cherry juice. The juice should half-cover the pears and ginger. Cover and simmer over low heat, until the pears are soft but not mushy, about 5 minutes, piercing with a toothpick to test for doneness. Remove the pears from the pot, reserving the juice, and transfer the pears to individual serving plates. Add the dissolved kudzu to the simmering juice and stir over low heat until thickened, 3 to 5 minutes. Pour 1 cup of the sauce over each pear and garnish with a mint sprig.

HOT AND COLD DRINKS

Rosemary Lemon Water

YIELDS 4 CUPS

- 1 quart filtered water
- 4 slices lemon
- 3 large sprigs rosemary, rinsed

Combine all the ingredients in a glass pitcher or jar and refrigerate for up to 8 hours. The rosemary will infuse the water almost immediately; leave the sprig in longer for stronger flavor.

Apple Ginger Tea

SERVES 1

- ½ cup green tea
- ½ cup apple juice
- ½-inch-long piece fresh ginger

Heat the green tea and apple juice in a saucepan over medium-low heat. Juice the ginger by passing through a garlic press and add to the tea. Serve immediately.

Pellegrino and Bitters Cocktail

Bitters is an herbal concentrate with a bitter flavor known to improve digestion. Its common ingredients are cascarilla, cassia, gentian, orange peel, and quinine. SERVES 1

12 ounces Pellegrino or other mineral water

1 teaspoon bitters (Angostura, Suze, or Peychaud's Bitters)

Lemon twist (optional)

Combine the Pellegrino and bitters and enjoy over ice or with a twist of lemon.

Gingered Green Tea

Green tea naturally contains some caffeine. Buy decaffeinated green tea if you prefer. Ginger is a gentle remedy for upset stomach and is warming on cold mornings. SERVES 1

1 green teabag

1 cup hot filtered water

1/2-inch-long piece fresh ginger, sliced

Place the teabag in a mug of hot water with 2 to 3 slices of ginger and serve.

Cinnamon Cider

This slightly more exotic version of hot apple cider has subtle flavors of India and a hint of maple. SERVES 2

2 cups unsweetened apple cider or apple juice

1/4 teaspoon ground cinnamon

1/4 teaspoon ground ginger

2 teaspoons maple syrup

1/2 orange, sliced

1/4 teaspoon ground cardamom (optional)

Fresh, peeled ginger slices (optional)

In a saucepan, heat the apple cider over low heat. Add the cinnamon, ginger, and maple syrup to the cider. Place the orange slices in 2 mugs and add the cardamom and fresh ginger. Pour the hot cider into the mugs and serve hot.

Citrus Sparkle

Use bottled sparkling water without additives or chemicals such as Calistoga mineral water or Perrier. SERVES 2

2 sweet citrus fruits such as orange or pink grapefruit

2 cups sparkling mineral water

Use a paring knife to remove the outer colored part of the fruit peel and be sure to leave the white pithy inner layer intact, because it is rich in bioflavonoids. Puree in a blender until smooth, mix with the mineral water, and serve immediately.

Cucumber and Lemon Water (Indian Springs Health Elixir)

This light refreshing drink is so tasty you'll be inspired to drink water all day long.

YIELDS 1 GALLON

1 cucumber, peeled and cored

1 lemon, sliced

1 gallon purified water or mineral water

Cut the cucumber into 4 long strips and place in a glass pitcher with the lemon slices. Cover with water and ice if desired. The cucumber and lemon will last all day. After you finish drinking the water, just add more to the pitcher.

Hibiscus Tea Cooler

This drink is light and only slightly sweet and can be made with a variety of juices.

SERVES 2

1 hibiscus teabag

1 cup hot water

1 cup cranberry juice

Steep the teabag in the hot water until the desired potency. Chill the tea in the refrigerator or add ice to cool. Combine with the cranberry juice and serve.

Apple Lemon Spritzer

SERVES 2

1 lemon or lime

2 apples

2 cups sparkling mineral water

Lemon wedges, for serving

Use a paring knife to remove the outer colored part of the lemon peel and be sure to leave the white pithy inner layer intact, because it is rich in bio-flavonoids. Add the apple and lemon to your juicer and juice according to the manufacturer's instructions. Pour into glasses with the mineral water and serve with lemon wedges.

SMOOTHIES

Smoothies are a creative and nourishing way to support your detoxification. Here are some tasty combinations to help you get started. You can also customize smoothies to fit your nutritional needs and taste. We have included a list of ingredient options on pages 246 and 247 to help you find the right combination to provide energy and nutrients while you satisfy your desire for sweet flavor in a balanced way. Smoothies can also be added to the Detox Diet for those who want to support their weight.

Ginger Cooler

SERVES 1

1 apple, cored, peeled, and sliced

$1/2$ cup filtered water

$1/2$ cup ice

1 lemon, peeled, halved, and seeded

2-inch-long piece fresh ginger, crushed

Combine all the ingredients in a blender and drink immediately.

Peachy Orange

SERVES 1

1 cup orange juice

1 cup fresh peaches or drained canned peaches

2 tablespoons vanilla protein powder

1 teaspoon nutritional yeast

Greens powder or flaxseed oil (optional)

Combine all the ingredients in a blender and drink immediately.

Strawberry-Orange Shake

SERVES 1

1 cup orange juice

1 cup frozen organic strawberries

1 frozen organic banana

200 mg vitamin C powder, protein powder, greens powder, or flaxseed oil (optional)

Combine all the ingredients in a blender and drink immediately.

Purple Papaya

SERVES 1

1 cup purple grape juice

1 cup fresh or frozen papaya slices

Protein powder, greens powder, or flaxseed oil (optional)

Combine all the ingredients in a blender and drink immediately.

Banana Soother

SERVES 1

- 1 cup rice milk
- 1 frozen organic banana
- 4 mint leaves
- Protein powder, greens powder, or flaxseed oil (optional)

Combine all the ingredients in a blender and drink immediately.

Avocado Freeze

SERVES 1

- $\frac{1}{2}$ avocado, peeled, pitted, and sliced
- 1 tablespoon freshly squeezed lemon juice
- 1 cup frozen cherries, pitted
- 1 cup orange juice
- Protein powder, greens powder, or flaxseed oil (optional)

Combine all the ingredients in a blender and drink immediately.

Tahini Shake

SERVES 2

- 1 cup rice milk
- 1 cup orange juice
- 1 frozen organic banana
- 2 tablespoons tahini
- Protein powder, greens powder, or flaxseed oil (optional)

Combine all the ingredients in a blender and drink immediately.

Cinnamon Pears

SERVES 2

- 2 pears, peeled and cored (or use canned pears)
- $\frac{1}{2}$ cup orange juice
- 1 teaspoon ground cinnamon
- Protein powder, greens powder, or flaxseed oil (optional)

Combine all the ingredients in a blender and drink immediately.

Tobin's Strawberry Almond Shake

SERVES 1

- $\frac{1}{2}$ cup almond milk
- $\frac{1}{2}$ cup organic frozen strawberries
- 2 tablespoons maple syrup

Combine all the ingredients in a blender and drink immediately.

SMOOTHIE INGREDIENT OPTIONS

- **Avocados**—The avocado is one of the richest plant sources of glutathione, a potent antioxidant that can detoxify environmental pollutants. It also contains vitamin E, another antioxidant, and enough oil to ensure that this fat-soluble vitamin is absorbed.

- **Beneficial microflora**—Acidophilus and Bifidus are two well-known organisms that are an important part of a healthy gut flora. Hundreds of similar organisms have now been identified that function in our intestines to help us digest our food completely, absorb natural beneficial hormones from plants, and fight off bad bacteria and viruses. Primal Defense (Garden of Life product) and other microflora replacement powders can be purchased at health food stores, grocery stores, and many pharmacies.

- **Brewer's yeast**—Nutritional yeast or brewer's yeast can be added to smoothies in small amounts without altering the flavor drastically. Add 1 teaspoon of either yeast powder to a smoothie to add folic acid, pyridoxine (vitamin B_6), and vitamin B_{12}.

- **Chlorella**—This blue-green algae is used in the detoxification of heavy metals such as cadmium, uranium, and lead. Studies in Japan have shown that chlorella increases the excretion of cadmium from people with cadmium poisoning. Chlorella contains many nutrients, especially amino acids, which support mental and physical energy and detoxification. Powdered chlorella is available at health food stores; Sun Chlorella is the most common brand. Start by adding just 1 teaspoon to your smoothies and then add more if you like the flavor.

- **Greens powders**—These are generally made of various algaes and chlorophyll (from barley grass or wheatgrass, for example), which provide minerals, trace minerals, and antioxidants to help remove free radicals from your body. Radiant Greens (G & W product), Perfect Food (Garden of Life product), ProGreens (Nutricology), Barleans Greens, and Green Vibrant are some brands on the market.

- **Milk alternatives**—Grain, bean, and nut milks can be used in place of dairy milk. There are many available in stores, such as oat milk, rice milk, almond milk, hazelnut milk, soy milk, multi-grain milk, hemp milk, and so forth. These products are sold in cartons and in aseptic boxes that do not require refrigeration. There are many varieties, such as vanilla, chocolate, low-fat, and organic. Buy organic to make sure the product is free of agricultural chemicals, and avoid the ones with flavor added because they are generally higher in sugar than their plain counterparts.

- **Nut butters**—Peanut butter, which is ground peanuts, is just one of the many nut butters. Cashew butter, almond butter, hazelnut butter, and even pistachio butter are now available. Buy high-quality nut butters without sugar, preservatives, or hydrogenated oils. Maranatha and Kettle are two brands that are of good quality.

- **Protein powders**—The protein in these powders is often from soybeans, which means you should look for organic soy protein powder; if that is not available, then look for non-GMO on the label. Non-GMO (genetically modified organism) indicates that the product is not genetically engineered. If you tolerate dairy, whey powders are popular and widely available. Rice and hemp seed proteins are also available in many stores.

- **Psyllium and chia seeds**—Psyllium seed is a rich source of soluble fiber called mucilage. The mucilage in psyllium seed aids in colon health, prevents constipation, and binds cholesterol and toxins in the intestine.

When added to water, psyllium seed powder can swell to ten times its original size. It is odorless and bland in taste but has a gritty texture that is reduced by adding it to a drink containing frozen fruit. Start with 1 teaspoon of psyllium seed powder and gradually work up to 1 tablespoon, to avoid developing gas. Drink a lot of water when you consume psyllium. Chia seeds are being used more for fiber support and they also contain some good fatty acids and are soothing to the GI tract.

- **Soluble fiber**—Psyllium seed powder, flaxseed powder, oat bran, and pectin are all soluble fiber sources that can be added to smoothies. Start with 1 teaspoon, working gradually up to 1 tablespoon. Soluble fiber is a type of carbohydrate that resists digestion by gastrointestinal secretions. It dissolves in the watery contents of the small intestine, producing a viscous gel. Soluble fiber binds with toxins in the colon. It also prevents constipation and lowers cholesterol levels.

Adapted from *Smoothies for Life!* by Daniella Chace and Maureen Keane (Prima Publishing, 1998).

Carrot Cocktail

SERVES 1

4 carrots

Handful of spinach

Handful of parsley

$1/2$ apple

Place all the ingredients in your juicer and juice according to the manufacturer's instructions. Serve immediately.

After Workout Refresher

SERVES 1

4 carrots

2 stalks celery

1 apple

Handful of parsley

Place all the ingredients in your juicer and juice according to the manufacturer's instructions. Serve immediately.

Energizing Elixir

SERVES 1

2 slices pineapple, with skin

$1/2$ cucumber

$1/2$ apple, seeded

Place all the ingredients in your juicer and juice according to the manufacturer's instructions. Serve immediately.

Cucumber Cooler

SERVES 1

1 lemon wedge (optional)

1 cucumber

1 apple

2 stalks celery

Use a paring knife to remove the outer colored part of the lemon peel and be sure to leave the white pithy inner layer intact. Place all the ingredients in your juicer and juice according to the manufacturer's instructions. Serve immediately.

Immune Supporter

SERVES 1

3 broccoli florets

1 clove garlic

4 carrots

Handful of spinach

Place all the ingredients in your juicer and juice according to the manufacturer's instructions. Serve immediately.

Apple Lemonade

You can add cucumber or celery to this recipe to increase the electrolytes. Any apple variety will be delicious in this juice combination, but Fuji apples are exceptionally tasty. SERVES 1

3 apples

$^1/_2$ lemon

Place all the ingredients in your juicer and juice according to the manufacturer's instructions. Serve immediately.

Tropical Twist

Lime juice over fresh papaya slices is a wonderful treat and just as tasty in this juice. SERVES 1

1 lime wedge

1 papaya, peeled

$^1/_4$-inch-long slice fresh ginger

Use a paring knife to remove the outer colored part of the lime peel and be sure to leave the white pithy inner layer intact. Place all the ingredients in your juicer and juice according to the manufacturer's instructions. Serve immediately.

Fresh Harvest

SERVES 1

2 cloves garlic

Handful of greens (kale, collards, spinach, and so on)

1 tomato

2 stalks celery

Place all the ingredients in your juicer and juice according to the manufacturer's instructions. Serve immediately.

Sunset Soother

SERVES 1

1 lemon wedge

1 cup cherries

1 bunch grapes

Use a paring knife to remove the outer colored part of the lemon peel and be sure to leave the white pithy inner layer intact. Place all the ingredients in your juicer and juice according to the manufacturer's instructions. Serve immediately.

Resources

Other Books by Dr. Elson Haas

Staying Healthy with Nutrition: The Complete Guide to Diet and Nutritional Medicine (Berkeley: Celestial Arts, 1992, updated 2006) with Buck Levin, PhD, RD. The definitive resource for understanding the significant role of nutrition in our health, it is used as a school textbook and home reference guide.

Staying Healthy with the Seasons (Berkeley: Celestial Arts, 1981, updated 2003). Dr. Haas's popular first book integrates Eastern and Western health systems with practical guidelines for nutrition, herbology, and exercise.

A Cookbook for All Seasons (Berkeley: Celestial Arts, 1995, not in print) with Eleonora Manzolini. Offers expert guidelines for a healthy transition from the Detox Diet with menu plans attuned to the seasons and more than 150 recipes.

Vitamins for Dummies (Foster City, CA: IDG Books Worldwide, 1999) with Christopher Hobbs.

The False Fat Diet (New York: Ballantine, 2001) with Cameron Stauth. A guide for practitioners and patients on food reactions and weight.

You may contact Dr. Elson Haas:
    haashealthonline.com
    pmcmarin.com
    Preventive Medical Center of Marin
    25 Mitchell Boulevard, Suite 8
    San Rafael, CA 94903
    415-472-2343 (phone)
    email: emhaas@sonic.net

Other Books by Daniella Chace

More Smoothies for Life (New York: Clarkson Potter, 2007). Contains 150 smoothie recipes designed to cure common ailments, increase longevity, and satisfy cravings with fat-burning snacks.

Smoothies for Life! (New York: Clarkson Potter, 1998) with Maureen Keane. This book contains smoothies recipes designed to improve energy, build endurance, burn fat, boost immunity, reduce stress, and more.

What to Eat If You Have Cancer (Chicago: Contemporary Books, 1996, updated 2006) with Maureen Keane. This nutrition plan is designed to help starve cancer cells while strengthening the body against disease and the rigors of treatment.

The What to Eat If You Have Cancer Cookbook (Chicago: Contemporary Books, 1997) with Maureen Keane. This cookbook companion to *What to Eat If You Have Cancer* features recipes that stress healthy and enjoyable eating, while addressing malnutrition and other side effects of cancer therapy.

What to Eat If You Have Heart Disease (Chicago: Contemporary Books, 1998) with Maureen Keane. A comprehensive guide to nutritional therapy for the various forms of cardiovascular disease.

The What to Eat If You Have Heart Disease Cookbook (Chicago: Contemporary Books, 2000) with Maureen Keane. A program for those interested in helping to combat heart disease through nutritional therapy, with delectable recipes.

What to Eat If You Have Diabetes (New York: McGraw-Hill, 1998, updated 2006).

The What to Eat If You Have Diabetes Cookbook (New York: McGraw-Hill, 1999) with Maureen Keane. Contains easy and delicious recipes for stabilizing blood sugar.

About the Authors

Elson M. Haas, MD

Dr. Elson Haas is an integrative, family medicine physician for nearly forty years and is Founder/Director of Preventive Medical Center of Marin in San Rafael, CA (founded 1984, www.pmcmarin.com). He is also the author of many books and articles in the areas of health, nutrition, and detoxification. Dr. Haas speaks nationally, and has also created new multimedia educational entertainment products (books, musical CD, and apps) for young children and families (www.seasonsstudios.com). Visit www.haashealthonline.com.

Daniella Chace

Daniella Chace, MSN, is a clinical nutritionist and author of twenty books on health and nutrition. She is the creator of the NAI NutriSigns nutrition signage program for grocery stores and the innovator behind the iEat for Life suite of iPhone and Netbook applications that provide medical nutrition guidance for those living with health conditions. She lives in Port Townsend, Washington. Visit www.daniellachace.com and www.nutritionistapproved.com.

Measurement Conversion Charts

Volume

U.S.	Imperial	Metric
1 tablespoon	$1/2$ fl oz	15 ml
2 tablespoons	1 fl oz	30 ml
$1/4$ cup	2 fl oz	60 ml
$1/3$ cup	3 fl oz	90 ml
$1/2$ cup	4 fl oz	120 ml
$2/3$ cup	5 fl oz ($1/4$ pint)	150 ml
$3/4$ cup	6 fl oz	180 ml
1 cup	8 fl oz ($1/3$ pint)	240 ml
$1 1/4$ cups	10 fl oz ($1/2$ pint)	300 ml
2 cups (1 pint)	16 fl oz ($2/3$ pint)	480 ml
$2 1/2$ cups	20 fl oz (1 pint)	600 ml
1 quart	32 fl oz ($1 2/3$ pints)	1 liter

Length

Inch	Metric
$1/4$ inch	6 mm
$1/2$ inch	1.25 cm
$3/4$ inch	2 cm
1 inch	2.5 cm
6 inches ($1/2$ foot)	15 cm
12 inches (1 foot)	30 cm

Temperature

Fahrenheit	Celsius/Gas Mark
250°F	120°C/gas mark $1/2$
275°F	135°C/gas mark 1
300°F	150°C/gas mark 2
325°F	160°C/gas mark 3
350°F	180 or 175°C/gas mark 4
375°F	190°C/gas mark 5
400°F	200°C/gas mark 6
425°F	220°C/gas mark 7
450°F	230°C/gas mark 8
475°F	245°C/gas mark 9
500°F	260°C

Weight

U.S./Imperial	Metric
$1/2$ oz	15 g
1 oz	30 g
2 oz	60 g
$1/4$ lb	115 g
$1/3$ lb	150 g
$1/2$ lb	225 g
$3/4$ lb	350 g
1 lb	450 g

Index

C

Cabbage
    Caraway Cabbage Borscht, 232–33
    Island Coleslaw, 105
    juice, 60
Caesarless Salad, 227
Caffeine
    case study of, 191
    detoxification from, 191–93, 195–96
    detox summary for, 196, 198
    drugs, 189, 193
    effects of, 188–89, 190–91, 194
    sources of, 186, 187, 189, 192–93
    supplements and, 192–93, 195, 197
    withdrawal symptoms, 188, 189
    See also Coffee
Calcium, 78
Cancer
    detoxification and, 123
    fasting and, 45, 49–50
    smoking and, 146, 147, 152, 154, 156
    sugar and, 132, 133
Candida albicans, 17, 33, 34, 133, 136
Caramelized Onion Quinoa, 235
Caraway Cabbage Borscht, 232–33
Carbohydrates
    diets low in, 143
    simple vs. complex, 91–92
Carrots
    After Workout Refresher, 248
    Carrot Cocktail, 248
    Carrot Smoothie, 71
    Immune Supporter, 248–49
    Island Coleslaw, 105
    juice, 60
    Lemon Veggie Delight, 72
Cascara sagrada, 79
Cayenne pepper, 50, 79
Celery juice, 60
Chai Cocoa, 103
Chaparral, 79
Chemicals
    cleaning without, 216
    clothing free of, 215–16
    in food, 27, 28, 91
    reducing exposure to, 129–30
    smoking and, 150
    See also Drugs
Cherries
    Avocado Freeze, 245

Cherry Ice, 103
    juice, 60
    Sunset Soother, 249
Cherry Tomato Salad and Ginger Dressing, 227
Chewing, 31, 36
Chia seeds, 80, 247
Children
    alcohol and, 170
    detoxification and, 118–19
    obesity in, 118–19
    smoking and, 147, 148, 156
    sugar and, 135–36, 144–45
Chlorella, 246
Chromium, 144
Chutney, Date and Orange, 237
Cider, Cinnamon, 242
Cigarettes. *See* Nicotine; Smoking
Cilantro
    Cilantro Guacamole, 105
    Cilantro Pesto, 238
Cinnamon
    Cinnamon Cider, 242
    Cinnamon Pears, 245
Citrobacter sp., 33
Citrus
    Citrus Sparkle, 242
    juice, 60
    See also individual fruits
Cleaning products, nontoxic, 211–12, 216
Cleansing. *See* Detoxification
Clothing, chemical-free, 215–16
Clover blossoms, red, 79
Cobalamin, 158
Cocaine, 207
Cocoa, Chai, 103
Coffee
    annual consumption of, 186
    caffeine in, 192
    decaffeinated, 186–87
    substitutes for, 195, 196
    transitional diets and, 91
    See also Caffeine
Cold Almonds, 239
Colds, 205
Coleslaw, Island, 105
Collard green juice, 60
Colon cleansing, 56–57, 75, 77
Colonoscopy, 33
Congestion
    diet and, 20–21
    problems related to, 7, 14
    symptoms of, 43
Constipation, 205

COPD (chronic obstructive pulmonary disease), 147, 153
Cotton, 215–16
Cousens, Gabriel, 42
Creamy Garlic Sauce, 237
Crohn's disease, 33
Cucumbers
    Asian Cucumber Salad, 234
    Cucumber and Lemon Water (Indian Springs Health Elixir), 243
    Cucumber Cooler, 248
    Energizing Elixir, 248
    Gazpacho, 231
    juice, 60
Cutting boards, 214
L-cysteine, 39, 78, 159

D

Dairy products
    alternatives to, 91, 246
    Glycemic Index of, 141
    organic, 90
Dandelion root, 79
Dani's Muesli, 226
Date and Orange Chutney, 237
Deficiency, symptoms of, 7
Dehydration, 81
Detox Diet
    benefits of, 63–64
    daily menu plan for, 67–68
    supplements for, 76
    for teenagers, 111
    transitioning from, 86
    See also Recipes
Detoxification
    best time for, 22–23, 26
    body's systems for, 11–12
    case studies of, 16–17, 22
    for children, 118–19
    controversy surrounding, 3–5
    definition of, 14
    determining need for, 8–9
    for elders, 121–22
    emotional challenges of, 12, 124, 126
    excessive, 12
    gallbladder and, 127
    herbs and, 79, 82
    importance of, 13–15
    individualizing program for, 19, 64–67
    levels of dietary, 15, 18, 19
    liver and, 126–27
    location for, 23, 26
    for men, 119–20
    mental, 12